BodySculpture

Plastic Surgery of the Body
For Men & Women

Alan M. Engler, M.D.

**HUDSON
PUBLISHING**

New York

This book is provided for educational and informational purposes only. It is not intended to be, and should not be used as, a replacement for appropriate medical and/or surgical care, nor is it intended to be a standard of care.

Published by:
Hudson Publishing
122 East 64th Street
New York, NY 10021

For more information, please visit www.bodysculpture.com

Printed in the United States of America

Publisher's Cataloging-in-Publication

Engler, Alan M.
    BodySculpture : plastic surgery of the body for men and
    women / Alan M. Engler. -- 2nd ed.
    p. cm.
    ISBN: 0-9663827-4-9

    1. Surgery, Plastic.   I. Title.

RD118.E64 1998   617.9'5
                                    QBI00-393

Dedication

This book is dedicated with love and gratitude to Danielle, Jeff, Steven, and the rest of my family, and to Bernadette, Doreen, and Barbara.

Acknowledgments

I gratefully acknowledge and thank the people who spent time reading drafts of this book, making corrections and suggestions, and discussing them with me: Danielle, Elizabeth Cheong, M.D., Arthur Cohen, Bernadette Ellinger, Janet Carlson Freed, Elizabeth Karcher, Carol Libby, Catherine Maniscalco, Barbara Salant, Berish Strauch, MD, and Mark Sultan, M.D. Their generous contributions are invaluable. I also thank Lexington Labs (New York) for the production of the photographs, Jaydee Camera Exchange, Inc., (New York), and my attorney, Robert Gold.

The illustrations were drawn by Li-Guo Liang, the Coordinator of Medical Illustrations in the Department of Plastic and Reconstructive Surgery, Albert Einstein College of Medicine, Bronx, New York. I thank him, as well as Han-Liang Yu, M.D., Assistant Professor and Director of the Division of Scientific Text and Visual Arts, for their assistance in the production of these illustrations.

Table of Contents

Preface

Over the past century or so a number of strikingly effective cosmetic surgery procedures have been developed, and they continue to undergo refinements and improvements. Advances in surgical techniques, instrumentation, and conceptual approaches have resulted in procedures that are safer, more effective, and more predictable than ever before. Increased popularity and acceptance, as well as market forces, have made these procedures, once the exclusive domain of only a small percentage of the population, widely available around the world. The goal of this book is to provide an overview of some of the most popular plastic surgery procedures of the body. It is not intended to be exhaustive and encyclopedic, or to cover every procedure that could be or has ever been used.

There is usually more than one way to do something, and different procedures and techniques can be equally effective. Furthermore, no two plastic surgeons do things exactly the same way. Except where otherwise noted, the statements in this book are my own and are derived from my training, experience, reading, and discussions with other surgeons. The conclusions drawn represent my personal preferences and are not presented as the only ways to accomplish the desired results.

The decision to undergo cosmetic surgery is highly individual. What is acceptable for one person may not be for someone else; big for one person is small for another. Because of its tendency to draw on people's insecurities and their desire to be told what they want to hear, plastic surgery lends itself particularly well to catchwords and slick marketing. Things are presented as black and white when there are actually many shades of gray. Existing procedures are rehashed and offered as new ones, and new procedures are routinely termed revolutionary. Anyone interested in plastic surgery should be, for his or her own benefit, educated, questioning, and wary. If something sounds too good to be true, it may be.

Sometimes it's not clear who's driving whom. The three M's of plastic surgery — marketing, media, and manufacturers — combine to recontour the plastic surgery landscape continuously, and sometimes quite rapidly. Doctors are as likely to be pulled into the wave of an innovation as to be leading it. Technological advances can be transformed from experimental to mainstream almost overnight. They may be abandoned just as quickly. New technologies may have side effects or consequences that do not become apparent for months and years. Plastic surgery is not the only field that is influenced by these forces, but because of its position at the crossroads of health and beauty, it is particularly susceptible to them.

Anybody considering cosmetic surgery, whether for him or herself, or for someone else, should do careful research. It is in this manner that this book can be useful — to provide information before a consultation with a qualified plastic surgeon, to serve as a reminder afterwards, and to be used as a general reference. It is meant to enhance a consultation, not to replace it. Because it discusses medical information, future developments may invalidate or require modification of the statements made in this book.

Introduction

The procedures described in this book are all elective procedures; that is, they are not emergencies. Furthermore, they don't have to be done at all. Most forms of surgery, even if elective, are things that need to be done for medical reasons; that is not the case for cosmetic surgery. Why, then, would anyone go through this? After all, cosmetic surgery may be cosmetic, but it is still surgery. One might think that elective surgery is not something people would rush to. And yet, they do — lots of them. Each year, hundreds of thousands of cosmetic surgery procedures are performed in the United States alone, and many times that around the world.

There are many possible explanations for this. Some are explored in this book, but the bottom line is that these procedures work. They can do things that nothing else can, i.e., effect a permanent change in specific parts of one's body. Not only that, but the patient gets to pick which part or parts are altered. That is demonstrated here, in words and photographs.

This book is divided into five sections: General Information, Breast Surgery, Liposuction, Tummy Tucks, and Results. The first section contains information that is common to most of the procedures, including preparation and things to know before surgery, anesthesia, what the day of surgery is like, the early recovery period, getting used to your new body, and long-term effects. A chapter entitled "Consequences and Complications" addresses, in a general sense, some of the things that can go wrong with plastic surgery.

The second section, Breast Surgery, discusses both breast enlargement and breast reduction. Breast enlargement is, literally, an enlargement of the existing breasts. This is done by inserting implants, of which there are many types, beneath the breast tissue. There are also different surgical techniques by which this can be accomplished. The other part of this section is entitled "Breast Lifts and Reductions." These procedures are put together because they are essentially the same operation. The differentiating factor (i.e., what constitutes a lift versus a reduction) is the amount of breast tissue that is removed. By one definition, if less than about 300 grams per side (about ten ounces) is removed, it is considered a "lift"; more than that is a "reduction."

The third section addresses liposuction, which is now the most commonly performed cosmetic surgery in the United States. While precise statistics are difficult to obtain, thousands of liposuctions are performed annually. Its popularity is understandable — it is a remarkably effective procedure. The details of liposuction are discussed, including how and why it works, surgical techniques, and what the recovery is like.

The fourth section discusses the treatment of the stomach when liposuction alone is not adequate. This refers to patients who have an excess of skin in one or more regions of the stomach. Almost all patients in this category have an excess of skin below the belly button (umbilicus); many also have an excess above it. Depending on the relative amounts and locations of excess skin and fat, and on how loose the abdominal muscles are, different treatments are indicated.

Finally, a photo gallery. These unretouched before-and-after photographs of my patients demonstrate some of the results that can be achieved with these procedures. Signed releases were obtained from all patients whose photos appear in this book.

Section 1
General Information

CHAPTER 1

"If they're pretty, you know they're smart"[1]

People like to look good, and most people want to look as good as they can. Much of our physical appearance is due to heredity and many aspects of the way we look are out of our control. Height, body frame, and the color of our eyes and hair are among the features that cannot, at present, be permanently altered. Many things, however, can be controlled. It is widely accepted that it makes sense to eat a healthful diet and to exercise. People who are truly concerned about their appearance adhere reasonably well to various regimens of diet and exercise. In order to optimize their appearance, people wear flattering clothes and jewelry, have their hair styled and colored a certain way, and use makeup. Some people go through all this for their own benefit (i.e., what they see in the mirror), some do it for others and most do it for both. Whether for personal and/or professional reasons, looking one's best can be a never-ending project.

In this society, as well as others, youth and beauty are considered desirable and attractive. People may wish that it were not so and may choose to ignore it, but it seems to be a fact, particularly in this day and age. Beauty is defined quite differently in different cultures and at varying times within the same culture. Contrast, for instance, the ample Rubenesque beauty of the seventeenth century with the waifish Twiggy look of the 1960s.

The explanation for this quest for beauty is controversial. While environmental or societal pressures and influence are

---

[1] From ABC News *20/20* report quoted in this chapter.

important factors, there is at least some suggestion that it originates from something more innate and instinctual. Beauty is an advantage throughout the animal kingdom. What we consider beautiful is often more notable in the male of the species than in the female (e.g., a lion's mane, or a peacock's feathers). Individuals with the most impressive arrays often win battles for territory and mates. There are other factors in these displays, such as the strength and superiority that such beauty may imply among animals, but beauty as a component of desirability is certainly not limited to humans.

Regardless of the basis of our interest in beauty, it has some tangible ramifications. Studies have shown repeatedly that attractive people are more likely to be successful, regardless of the standard used. Better jobs, more effective salespeople, more money. This is true for both men and women.

One report in which this phenomenon was demonstrated convincingly aired on ABC News' *20/20* (Friday, November 4, 1994, Transcript #1444). In one portion of this report, two people — one more attractive and one less attractive — were placed into a series of identical situations, such as job interviews. Make-up was used to exaggerate the differences, and certain standards of Western beauty were assumed. The people used for this test were actors. They were given identical resumes, clothes, etc., and were trained to say very little so as to let the interviewer take the lead. The results were striking and consistent, for both men and women. Prospective employers, as evidenced by hidden cameras as well as from interviews, repeatedly considered the attractive person to be more intelligent, more capable, and to have more potential than the less attractive person. Another test situation was a mock trial. In this case, prospective jurors were more likely to find the attractive "defendant" innocent, and when confronted with the two "defendants," they readily admitted that the overall appearance, including attractiveness and neatness, had been the deciding factor.

It's not just adults who respond in this manner. When the

two test subjects were "teachers," first graders thought that the more attractive people were better teachers. They consistently rated them as smarter, nicer, and as better storytellers. According to one first grader, "Teachers who look pretty are smart," and the title quote of this chapter came from another child. In a startling demonstration of how early these prejudices appear, one-year-old children (who typically withdraw from strangers) withdrew more from the plain faces than from the attractive ones. Even three-month-old babies spent more time staring at pictures of attractive faces than at less attractive ones. One might claim that adults just like to look at attractive people but don't want to admit it. Even if that's true, the argument for an exclusively societal origin to our preference for beauty weakens considerably as the age of the subject is lowered to the levels shown in this report.

It works the other way, too. Research has shown that pretty children get more attention from teachers than plain ones. Throughout life, attractive people are assumed to be warm, sensitive, kind, interesting, poised, and outgoing.[2]

It appears that in at least some situations there are advantages to being attractive. Of course, the beauty enhancers mentioned above are all temporary. Cosmetic surgery is permanent, which is an important distinction, but it accomplishes things that cannot be done any other way. This is not to claim that beauty, in and of itself, will necessarily provide happiness, make someone a "good" or kind person, or maintain or repair a relationship. Nevertheless, the powerful impact that beauty has in our daily lives, whether personal or professional, may help explain the popularity of plastic surgery. One might wonder if this phenomenon is just a sign of our times. Actually, while people want the most modern and up-to-date plastic surgery procedures, there's nothing new about our desire to look our best.

---

[2] *The New York Times.* October 26, 1997. Section 14, p 1.

CHAPTER 2

Plastic Surgery — Then and Now

Exactly how long people have been interested in cosmetic surgery is not known. Interest in creating a more youthful appearance, however, goes back a long way. An Egyptian hieroglyphic document from 1600 B.C. describes an ointment: "Anoint a man therewith. It is a remover of wrinkles from the head. When the flesh is smeared therewith it becomes a beautifier of the skin, a remover of blemishes, of all disfigurements, of all signs of age, of all weaknesses which are in the flesh. Found effective myriads of times." The precise makeup of this preparation is apparently unavailable, perhaps in part because the chief ingredient is the *hemayet* fruit, which is, at present, unidentified.[3] Evidently, interest in looking one's best and in reversing the effects of aging are not recent phenomena.

Through the ages many different "remedies" and interventions have been proposed to alter the appearance of specific body parts. Hemlock could supposedly prevent excessive breast growth (1558), and redundant eyelid skin could seemingly be removed by tightening metal screw-clamps and letting the skin fall off (1583). A century ago, a U.S. patent was issued for a device that purported to remove excess fat by rocking the offending portion of the body on the floor after the patient was strapped into a large metal contraption.[4] A seven-screwed metal clamp called the Nose Shaper Model Trados 25 was advertised as being able to produce the "Successful Correction of Ill-Shaped Noses for Men and Women."

[3] Hayes, H. Jr., (Ed.). *An Anthology of Plastic Surgery*, Rockville, MD, Aspen Publishers, Inc.,1986. page 13.
[4] Ibid pp 65, 138, and 175.

Although the first breast reduction may have been performed as early as A.D. 650, modern cosmetic surgery is generally felt to have emerged toward the end of the nineteenth century. The development of anesthesia (first general anesthesia, then local) made much of this possible. Many of the earliest surgeons were in or from Germany, including Erich Lexer (1867–1937), who pioneered modern breast reduction surgery. Experience with severe facial injuries during the First World War led to greater familiarity with surgery of the head and neck. Facial reconstructive procedures evolved into cosmetic surgery of the nose and the face. Among the earliest surgeons in this arena were Jacques Joseph and Gustave Aufricht, who helped develop nasal surgery, and Sir Harold Gillies, a British surgeon who described facial reconstruction by repositioning facial skin, later adapting it for use in cosmetic surgery.

Contrary to popular belief, the name "plastic surgery" does not come from the use of plastics in the surgery. While plastic materials (such as the silicone in breast implants) are used, the term plastic surgery was in use long before implants made of plastic were developed. Instead, plastic surgery refers to the strict definition of the word "plastic" — "capable of being molded or of receiving form."[5] Plastic is used in the sense of changing the position of skin, moving skin and tissue from one part of the body to another, stretching things out and shaping them. This meaning of plastic came to be used for the class of moldable, changeable materials that we now normally refer to as plastics, not the other way around.

The first breast implants in the modern era were developed in the 1950s. Silicone implants were reported by Thomas Cronin, in 1962. Many different materials have been used to increase the size of the breasts. In Asia, for example, women underwent injections of paraffin, often with disastrous results. The quest for the perfect breast implant material continues, which is discussed in subsequent chapters.

[5] *Webster's Encyclopedic Unabridged Dictionary*, New York, Gramercy Books, 1994.

Liposuction was developed in the 1960s and 1970s by, among others, a French surgeon, Yves Gerard Illouz, who adapted and improved techniques that had been introduced about fifty years earlier.

Regardless of its origins, plastic surgery is now firmly entrenched in our collective psyche. This is evidenced by a short trip to a newsstand or bookstore, or by "surfing" through television or radio stations. The pervasiveness of plastic surgery was underscored by an incident I inadvertently participated in several years ago.

On a hot August day I was walking through a department store. It was during a heat wave — the type where everyone is advised to stay indoors and seek shelter in a shopping mall if air conditioning is not available. As I headed for the exit I passed through the cosmetics department. Walking toward me was a woman in her 40s and a girl, presumably her daughter, about 15 years old. As they approached, I saw that the girl was becoming a bit wobbly on her feet. I moved nearer to them just as her eyes rolled back and she started to faint. I jumped forward, caught her as she was falling, and lowered her onto the ground. Her mother became hysterical and blurted out that her daughter hadn't eaten a thing for lunch. After determining that the girl had simply fainted and would be okay, I reassured her mother. I asked for some water. A store employee brought out an atomizer of designer water, which I sprayed onto the girl's face. She opened her eyes and looked up at the ceiling. Her mother, now calmed, turned to me and, noticing my beeper, asked if I was a doctor. I nodded. Next she asked what kind of doctor I was. "Actually," I said, "I'm a plastic surgeon." At that point the girl, apparently revived but still lying flat on her back, lifted her head up sharply and asked, "Oh wow! Do you do liposuction?" The mere mention of plastic surgery appears to have spurred her recovery.

Plastic surgery has also gained acceptance by men, a fact noted by, among others, *The Wall Street Journal.* [6] Men now

---

[6] *The Wall Street Journal.* August 28, 1991. page B1.

constitute about 15–20% of plastic surgery patients (and more in some practices), which is about double what it was fifteen years ago. Increasingly, men seem to have concluded that a more youthful appearance may increase their likelihood of success in the highly competitive business world, as well as benefit them personally. This is reflected in their interest in cosmetic surgery.

Despite its benefits, plastic surgery is not for everyone. Some people are plastic surgery "enthusiasts," and some aren't. Time has a way of changing one's perspective, however. More than one person nearing or in her 40s has confided that after years of insisting that she would never have plastic surgery, things might be different now. It's not necessarily a question of looking a decade or so younger (even though that might be nice), but rather of looking as good as one reasonably can.

Plastic surgery is a dynamic field. New developments appear on a regular basis and what is accurate now may not be so in the future. Better results can be produced using smaller incisions than ever before. Today's most popular procedures were essentially unknown several decades ago. This seems only fair: A field that is defined by "capable of being molded" should be expected to be modified itself on a regular basis.

CHAPTER 3

The Consultation

The consultation is the first step taken by the prospective patient. It is the time for the doctor and the patient to meet each other, and for the doctor to interview, examine, and assess the patient. Literature about the procedure(s) in question may be given to the patient at this time, if it has not been mailed out in advance. Photographs of other patients who have had the surgery in question are often shown: the before-and-after photos. At the conclusion, the doctor proposes a procedure or procedures that can produce the desired result. Of course, that depends to a great extent on what the patient wants.

With cosmetic surgery, realistic expectations are an integral part of the equation. It has been written that "all men are created equal."[7] With no disrespect intended, and noting that the quote does not come from a scientific text, some plastic surgeons might disagree. Bodies come in a wide range of shapes and sizes; like snowflakes, it appears that no two are the same. Not all things are possible for all bodies. It is as important to know what the procedures will not do as it is to know what they will do. Sometimes what one needs to hear most is what is not possible.

Consultations vary from office to office. Some include a detailed discussion with the doctor; others are conducted primarily by a trained administrator, physician's assistant, or nurse, with the doctor spending only a few minutes with the patient. They also vary in duration, with some lasting up to an hour and others only ten to fifteen minutes. Sometimes educational videos are shown. No single type of consultation is inherently more effective, accurate, or correct than any other.

The consultation is also the time for the patient to

---

[7] *The Declaration of Independence, 1776.*

interview the doctor. Patients tend to be quite knowledgeable about the procedures they're interested in. This benefits everyone, since a consultation is more productive when patients are at least somewhat "educated" beforehand, rather than trying to learn everything at a single office visit. There is a tremendous amount of information available and patients often bring with them, or have at home, a folder containing magazine articles, newspaper clippings, notes, and a list of questions. More recently, this has included information obtained from the Internet and other electronic media. This is not surprising since one does not typically schedule an appointment with a doctor the first time plastic surgery is considered. The process starts with being unhappy about, and then analyzing, one or more areas of one's body. It continues with reading about choices in magazines or newspapers, watching television and news reports, and having discussions with family, friends, co-workers, physicians, and beauty and/or hair salon personnel. The latter are often highly knowledgeable about plastic surgery, as their business concerns people's appearances. They typically see, among their customers, a wide range of procedures performed by different plastic surgeons within their communities, and for this reason, they are useful sources of information. Dermatologists, obstetricians, and gynecologists tend to be particularly good sources of referrals, although any doctor may have excellent suggestions. Recommendations can also be obtained from professional societies.

One of a surgeon's qualifications is his or her board certification status. A board is a group of doctors that seeks to establish and maintain certain professional standards. This is done by assessing a doctor's education, training, surgical expertise, and judgment. There are several different boards that incorporate or encompass plastic surgery. Once a surgeon has met the requirements of a board, he or she is termed "board-certified." Being board-certified does not guarantee a result and there are competent surgeons who are not board-certified. Nevertheless, it represents a certain level of achievement, and it is generally considered prudent to select a surgeon who is board-certified. There are now so many qualified surgeons who are board-certified that it is easier than ever to find one. Many patients will only choose a surgeon who is board-certified.

There are advantages and disadvantages to every surgical procedure. In many fields of surgery, the decisions are clear-cut: for example, a laceration that needs to be sutured. Plastic surgery, however, is different. Each procedure, from breast implants to reduction, from liposuctions to tummy tucks, is associated with certain features and characteristics that may be right for one person but not for another. Where options are available, it is normally preferable to choose those that are best in the long run. The surgical plan should be individualized for each patient, and the basis for accomplishing that is the information exchanged during the consultation.

The patient's medical history and any underlying medical problems, even those that seem insignificant, should be reviewed and discussed at the consultation. Certain medical conditions and habits may lead the doctor to alter his or her recommendations, or may preclude the surgery altogether. Once the proposed procedures have been discussed, the surgeon (or representative) discusses where they will be done, under what level of anesthesia or sedation, and what the typical recovery period is like. These topics are covered in subsequent chapters.

Another function of the consultation is to initiate informed consent. Informed consent is a term for the discussion the surgeon has with the patient about the proposed surgery, including its risks, benefits, and alternatives. The objective is to discuss the relevant information so that a "reasonable" person can decide whether or not to undergo the proposed surgery. The goal of informed consent is an ambitious one. It is not realistic to expect a surgeon, in one or more office visits, to transfer what he or she knows about the proposed surgery, both specifically and in context, to a lay person, and for that person to comprehend fully what has been discussed. Nevertheless, the intent is to come as close to that as is feasible. It is not possible to offer guarantees with surgical procedures.

Finally, the costs for the proposed procedure(s) are discussed. These may be presented as a single, global fee (encompassing the expenses for anesthesia, the facility, and any materials, such as implants), or each component may be listed separately. Fees and financial policies vary widely, not only in different parts of the country, but even within a given region. In some offices, the costs of the surgery are addressed at the beginning of the consultation, in others, near or at the end. Fees for cosmetic surgery are normally paid in advance of the surgery. Surgery is not identical from surgeon to surgeon, making precise comparisons difficult.

In summary, the initial consultation is the time for the patient to learn as much as possible about what, in that surgeon's opinion, would best accomplish what the patient wants. Many patients, relying on a referral from a satisfied patient or another source, use the consultation as a confirmation of what they have essentially already decided; sometimes they just want to know the price. Others, for educational, financial, and other reasons, have consultations with more than one surgeon. On the basis of the consultation(s), the patient makes a decision about the surgery, both whether or not to do it, and if so, when. Once the surgery is scheduled, more information is given, and routines and guidelines are discussed, but the first step is the consultation.

CHAPTER 4

Anesthesia

The goal of plastic surgery is an excellent result, but the primary concern is the safety of the patient. This starts with making sure that the patient does not have any underlying medical conditions that may affect the way anesthesia can be administered safely and extends to overseeing the entire procedure from a medical standpoint. The patient needs to be sedated and/or anesthetized appropriately; clearly, the procedure is performed most effectively when the anesthesia is administered correctly. Some procedures can be performed under local anesthesia alone (although even in these cases many patients prefer at least some sedation). For the procedures described in this book, anesthesia (literally, "lack of sensation") is complete; the patient does not feel pain during the procedure. Because of the sedation used, the patient is typically unaware of the surroundings and remembers that portion of the day as a blur, if at all.

The skill and experience of the anesthesiologist are key. Not all anesthesiologists are equally trained and adept at administering the anesthesia that is often used for plastic surgery. Most plastic surgeons have a few "favorite" anesthesiologists (physicians) or anesthetists (nurses). Both physicians and nurses can administer the anesthesia properly; the specific professional degree does not automatically confer expertise. Outpatient anesthesia is really a sub-specialty in its own right. An anesthesiologist (from here on this term will be used for both physicians and nurses) may be proficient in inpatient general anesthesia, but less capable at administering anesthesia designed for plastic surgery.

Anesthesia has its own risks. From airway and breathing

problems to blood pressure fluctuations and a wide range of reactions to the medications administered, the anesthesia is an essential but complex aspect of the surgical procedure. Its use is operator-dependent, and the skill of the anesthesiologist is that much more important with the newer medications that are powerful but short-acting.

Twenty years ago a discussion of anesthesia would have been simpler than it is today. Medications developed since then have blurred some of the distinctions between the types of anesthesia available. Previously, there were four major categories applicable to plastic surgery: general anesthesia, regional anesthesia, light sedation, and local anesthesia. General anesthesia is when the responsibility for breathing, pain relief, and sedation is taken over by someone, and something, other than the patient. This means inhalation anesthetics (gases administered by a machine) and, often, endotracheal intubation (i.e., a tube in the throat). Regional anesthesia numbs specific portions of the body and is often coupled with sedation. An example of this is an epidural block. Known most widely for its use during labor and delivery, it can be used for plastic surgery procedures of the lower body. The next choice is sedation, which consists of oral and/or intravenous agents, all of which were, originally, relatively long-acting. Ironically, the level of sedation they produced was light by today's standards. With all of these forms of anesthesia, nausea and disorientation, lasting up to several days postoperatively, were common. Finally, there is local anesthesia alone. With this form of anesthesia only the immediate area being operated upon is numbed; nothing else is administered, including drugs that might relax the patient and make him or her less aware of what is happening.

In the past few years, however, a new group of intravenous anesthetic agents have changed the way anesthesia can be administered. Some of these are entirely new drugs; others are similar to existing drugs. Although typically described as deep intravenous sedation, they can produce a level of anesthesia that is probably more accurately termed "intravenous general anesthesia." These agents are powerful but extremely short-acting: patients start to "wake up" just a few minutes after the medications are stopped. They are ideal for people who do not want traditional general anesthesia, since it seems like one is having local anesthesia with a little light sedation. As an added benefit, they have fewer and less severe side effects (such as nausea) than older medications.

These anesthetics are an enormous improvement over those that were previously available. This is illustrated by a man who underwent a liposuction of the chest (for gyneco-mastia — see Chapters 33 and 41) at 9:30 in the morning; two hours later he left the office with a friend and went out to lunch. Though not typical, this is virtually unheard of with any of the older forms of anesthesia (aside from local anesthesia alone).

As with the surgery itself, the anesthesia should be individualized. The procedure(s) being performed, as well as the preferences of the surgeon and the patient, are important factors in selecting the type and level of anesthesia. Some procedures mandate relatively deep anesthesia. Examples include large breast reductions, tummy tucks, and submuscular breast implants. Other procedures are routinely performed under lighter anesthesia or, in some cases, under local anesthesia alone. Regardless of what type or level is selected, the skillful administration of the anesthesia facilitates both the surgery and the recovery, making the entire experience safer and easier to tolerate.

CHAPTER 5

Where is the Surgery Performed?

Plastic surgery can be performed in several different types of facilities. The actual location used depends largely on the surgeon. Some surgeons operate exclusively (or nearly so) in an office-based or other free-standing surgical facility, some operate exclusively in hospitals (whether on an outpatient basis or with an overnight stay), and some operate in either environment. Some surgeons have such a good working relationship with a nearby hospital that it functions essentially like a private facility. Where a surgeon chooses to operate may depend on the procedure to be performed, with larger, longer, or more complicated procedures being done in a hospital. Sometimes it depends on the patient. Patients may prefer a specific location, or underlying medical conditions may mandate a hospital setting (although these patients are less likely to undergo elective plastic surgery). The choice of location for plastic surgery does not in itself guarantee or preclude any particular result or experience; it is usually a question of the surgeon's and/or the patient's preferences.

Financial considerations may be a factor, too. Plastic surgery procedures can often be performed more cost-effectively in an office or outpatient setting. The constant shifts in health care and the way hospitals are staffed, reimbursed, and provide care mean that all of these conditions are subject to change, even in the near future.

There are advantages and disadvantages of each of the types of facilities that can be used. Advantages of outpatient facilities include specialization toward plastic surgery procedures, privacy, and comfort (which are even more pronounced in office-based facilities). Disadvantages include the relative lack of support services and ancillary care (laboratories, X-rays, etc.). Advantages of hospital-based facilities include the proximity to other physicians and equipment, increased support services (such as waiting rooms and cafeterias), and ancillary care. Disadvantages include a more impersonal setting, more administrative requirements and paperwork, less specialization for plastic surgery, and association with patients (and their physicians) who are not undergoing elective plastic surgery. This can be uncomfortable if, for example, a patient in the hospital for cosmetic surgery shares a room or has prolonged contact with a patient who has a medical problem.

Increasingly, plastic surgery is performed on an ambulatory basis. After the surgery the patient returns to his or her home or hotel. Nurses or other attendants are available to assist the patient for one or more days following the surgery. Some surgeons have a recovery suite or hotel within or near their surgical facility. Patients may remain there for up to a week or more, recovering from the surgery in a wide range of accommodations. Some of these are in — or essentially are — luxury hotels, complete with spas, gourmet food, and lots of attentive care.

The procedures described in this book can be performed in any adequate surgical facility, including an office-based surgical suite, a free-standing ambulatory surgery center, or a traditional hospital, whether on an outpatient or inpatient basis. There are reasons why certain procedures may be best performed in one place or another, but from the standpoint of safety and results, no surgical facility is inherently superior to any other.

CHAPTER 6

The Day of Surgery (and Preparing for It)

Once the date of surgery is set, a routine is set into motion. Most offices provide booklets that guide the patient through this stage. Any medications that one takes are reviewed, including over-the-counter preparations. In general, for a period of three weeks before and after surgery, all non-essential medications and preparations should be discontinued. Some medications may need to be temporarily adjusted, altered, or eliminated after consulting with the prescribing physician. A number of these need to be avoided because they interfere with the normal blood-clotting system and can increase the risk of excessive bleeding, both during and after the surgery. These medications include aspirin, ibuprofen, Advil®, Motrin®, Nuprin®, Alleve®, etc. There are many prescription and non-prescription products that contain aspirin or compounds that have similar effects. Some seemingly harmless and beneficial substances, like Vitamin E, can increase the risk of bleeding. There are even some reports that garlic can have the same effect. Acetaminophen (e.g., Tylenol®), or products that exclusively use acetaminophen as a pain reliever, can normally be used safely during this period.

Different surgeons have different protocols. Some prefer to have their patients take certain vitamins; others endorse dietary programs and/or herbal supplements. Some habits, such as tobacco smoking, can affect the healing process, particularly for procedures like breast reductions, tummy tucks, and facelifts (see Chapters 21 and 34). There is relatively little standardization in preoperative regimens. About 7–10 days before surgery, blood (and other) tests are often done.

On the day of surgery, the patient typically arrives at the surgical suite or hospital in the morning or early afternoon. After registering, going into a room, and changing into a gown, he or she may then meet with the surgeon to go over the procedure one more time, to undergo markings for the proposed areas of surgery, and to discuss any last minute questions. Sometimes the patient does not meet with the surgeon until just before the surgery. Measurements, such as weight, hip and waist circumference, etc., may be taken. The surgical consent form is signed, if that has not already been done. Despite everything that may be discussed ahead of time, many of the most important decisions (e.g., precisely how much skin and/or fat is removed) are made during the surgery.

The patient is also interviewed by any nursing and anesthesia personnel. At this point, the patient may start taking some of the medications that provide sedation, such as one or more capsules or tablets; with other protocols, no oral medications are used. The patient is then taken into the Operating Room or a nearby area where an intravenous line is started (this may not be done if local anesthesia alone is being used). Shortly thereafter the first medications are administered. The patient usually remembers nothing from this point until sometime after the surgery has been completed. There is, effectively, a several hour gap in the patient's day. Antibiotics are often administered intravenously; sometimes they are taken orally starting one day before the surgery. Depending on the procedure, the actual operating time normally ranges from about 45 minutes to 5 hours.

At the completion of the surgery, bandages and/or a compression garment are applied. The garment may be a bra (for breast surgery), a girdle (for the thighs, or hips), a wrap-around velcro binder (stomach or chest), a vest (chest), or a chin-strap (face, neck). In some cases, the compression is fashioned with elastic tape or bandages. After a short period of recovery (up to several hours), the patient goes home or to a nearby hotel, accompanied by a relative, friend, or nurse (for ambulatory procedures), or is admitted to a hospital room (for inpatient procedures). Once they are awake enough (usually shortly after the surgery), patients are able to get up and walk at least a little bit. They are encouraged to do so since early ambulation has been shown to facilitate breathing and to decrease the likelihood of developing blood clots in the legs. Most patients go home, get into bed, and sleep through the night, awakening only to have something to eat or drink, and to go to the bathroom. In the case of tummy tucks and many procedures performed under general anesthesia, patients often remain in bed until the following morning.

The patient should be accompanied by a responsible adult for at least the first 24 hours after surgery. This is primarily for assistance in general, but is prudent after any surgery.

CHAPTER 7

The Early Recovery Period

The first night after surgery is often surprisingly mild. This is because the anesthesia used during surgery is combined with, or has effects like, long-acting analgesic (pain-relieving) medications. Over the next several days, the body eliminates these medications. Symptoms may increase during this time. Maximum swelling and bruising — and therefore discomfort — may not occur until 1–3 days after the surgery. When bruising starts out relatively deep (as after a liposuction), it may take longer to peak, e.g., 5–10 days.

Within a few days of the surgery most patients obtain adequate relief from postsurgical discomfort by using extra strength acetaminophen (Tylenol®), with occasional use of a stronger medication. Some patients never use anything other than Tylenol®. Oral medications are provided for pain relief and are used according to a schedule. Two or more levels of pain relievers are often supplied; if necessary, the stronger medication is used for the first few days, followed by the more moderate preparation. Excessive use of pain medications can be associated with a number of unpleasant side effects such as headaches, nausea, dizziness, and constipation.

Pain and pain perception vary widely. Some patients report relatively mild pain after their surgery while others, after the same procedure, report more. The degree of pain can be related to specific procedures. Some procedures are routinely associated with somewhat more pain (such as submuscular breast implants), others with less. Breast reductions, for example, are often associated with surprisingly little discomfort. Discomfort sometimes becomes more pronounced at night; this is partly a consequence of one's daytime activity, and partly because as one settles down for the evening there are fewer distractions and any discomfort is harder to ignore. Swelling, bruising, discoloration, itching, tingling, numbness, and asymmetry (e.g., one side different from the other) are common at this stage. Surgery can be exhausting, both physically and emotionally. Now is the time to rest, and to let the body heal. The doctor and office staff typically provide lots of support throughout this period.

The stitches are removed at one or more office visits over a period of days to weeks, depending on the procedure and the surgeon's preference. For the procedures described in this book, the first stitches are usually removed starting about one week after the surgery. Increasingly, absorbable (self-dissolving) stitches are used in many procedures, thereby eliminating the need for suture removal. In some cases (e.g., some liposuctions), no stitches are used. Office visits are scheduled for various times after the surgery for dressing (bandage) changes and to monitor the recovery.

The patient often has a larger role in the recovery than one might think. Among the most important factors is one's state of mind. Sometimes the recovery (like work!) seems to contract or expand to fill the available time. People who have plastic surgery tend to be relatively ambitious and energetic, which is to their advantage. Repeatedly, patients who come in determined to recover quickly from their surgery and return to work as rapidly as possible — are able to do exactly that. That is not an ironclad rule or a guarantee, just an observation. Conversely, patients convinced that they will have a difficult recovery seem to become enmeshed in a self-fulfilling prophecy. It is normal to be sore, uncomfortable and tired, and it may take a while to feel 100%. Often it's two steps forward, one step back — a good day or period is followed by a less good one. One patient said that the recovery is like childbirth: it's not exactly fun, but it's temporary, it fades from memory, and in any event, it's well worth it. What the recovery is like may be an issue of pain, pain tolerance, one's state of mind, and, perhaps even more so, what one doesn't mind. With plastic surgery, the power of positive thinking should not be underestimated.

CHAPTER 8

What Will the Neighbors Say?

The answer to this depends on other factors, among them, how much surgery was done and in which areas, what type of clothes did you wear before and what type of clothes do you wear now, do you tend to keep things to yourself or do you tell everybody everything (one of my patients said that, for months after her surgery, she would ask friends she hadn't seen in a while, "Which do you want to hear about first, my broken ankle or my liposuction?"), and finally, how observant are your neighbors?

In general, the most dramatic changes occur when the most surgery has been done. When the stomach, hips, and thighs have been recontoured by liposuction, one's clothing size can drop by several sizes; depending on the type of clothing worn, this can clearly be noticeable. On the other hand, if surgery was done only on the thighs and knees, and loose, below-knee skirts are worn both before and after surgery, then the changes will be concealed. Similarly, if one's breasts have been increased by two cup sizes from breast enlargement, it may be difficult to conceal it. Patients may or may not want to camouflage their new bodies; depending on the degree of what has been done, it may be nearly impossible to do so.

A typical scenario is illustrated by breast reduction surgery. After breast reductions, patients are often asked how they were able to lose 30 pounds so quickly (when less than five pounds of breast tissue was actually removed). There are at least two reasons for this. First, large breasts, particularly if associated with sagging, make people look heavier than they really are. This has to do with the overall impression one's body makes. Large breasts present an image of a shorter waist which, when compared with someone of identical height and weight but with a longer waist, makes a body look heavy. Secondly, people make an assumption, whether conscious or subconscious, about how much weight the person would have had to lose in order to look as good as he or she actually does.

The most common reaction from friends and neighbors who do notice a change tends to be something like, "Gee, you look good lately. Were you away?" or "Your clothes look great," or "Is your hair different?" People may know that something is different and that you look better, but they often can't figure out what it is. This happens with many plastic surgery procedures. After a facelift or eyelid surgery, comments may be no more specific than "You look great — you don't look as tired lately." After a liposuction, people may think that you lost some weight, concluding that all that dieting and exercising finally paid off and that the credit should go to your health club.

The specific improvement achieved by the surgery tends to be identified much less often than one might expect. In fact, to decrease even further the likelihood that the surgical alteration will be noticed, we often recommend getting exactly what other people think they're seeing — a new haircut, color or style, new glasses, and/or some new clothes. This strategy can deflect attention from the recently altered area(s), and allow one's family and friends (those who are not in the know) to become accustomed more gradually to the "renovated" shape.

Of course, a few people may figure out exactly what happened. Sometimes they know so much because they or someone they know well has had the same thing done; other times they're just well-informed, observant, and "onto" it. What you tell people is up to you. You can fool some of the people all of the time, and all of the people some of the time. Sometimes, you can even fool Mom.

CHAPTER 9

Consequences and Complications

The goal of any surgical procedure is a flawless operation, an uneventful recovery, and an excellent result. Most of the time that's what happens. Nevertheless, plastic surgery is surgery and, as such, is associated with the risk of certain complications. These are rare, and are minimized by the use of appropriate patient selection and good surgical judgment, technique, and aftercare. In most cases, early recognition and prompt treatment turn a potentially serious complication into a relatively minor disturbance. The best treatment, of course, is prevention.

A wide range of problems can occur with plastic surgery. Nearly everything imaginable has been reported to have happened as a result of, during, or after surgical procedures. It is not always possible to identify precisely why any specific problem occurred. An exhaustive and complete discussion of complications is beyond the scope of this publication.

There are some potential problems that are unique to each surgical procedure (these are detailed in subsequent chapters) and some that are common to all. Some of these typically become apparent early (i.e., within the first few hours or days after surgery), and some may not be evident for several weeks or months.

Early complications include bleeding problems, which can be either excessive bleeding or blood clot formation. Bleeding occurs to a limited degree with all surgical procedures. When bleeding is minimal, it is not medically worrisome; the body absorbs small amounts of blood routinely without adverse effects, (e.g., a bruise). Excessive bleeding can occur for a number of reasons. It can result from having taken certain medications, such as aspirin, ibuprofen, and related compounds, all of which "thin the blood" and increase the risk of bleeding. It can be associated with some cyclical conditions (the premenstrual period and several days immediately after the onset of menses, during which there may be total body swelling and increased bleeding). Excessive bleeding may occur if there are previously unknown bleeding disorders, or as a result of suboptimal control of bleeding at the time of surgery. It may also start up after the surgery, due to changes in blood pressure or for other reasons. Often the precise explanation for excessive bleeding during or after surgery remains unknown. Early recognition and prompt intervention are the keys to minimizing the long-term effects of a complication. Severe bleeding, for example, can mandate urgent reoperation, often within 24–48 hours of the first procedure. Blood clot formation in the lower legs and related problems are associated with prolonged immobility and inactivity. Early postoperative movement and ambulation markedly decrease the risk of this occurring.

Another potential complication is infection. Infections are often secondary to bleeding, although they can also occur without an obvious cause, particularly if a foreign body (like a breast implant) is used. Infections are usually treated with antibiotics, with or without irrigation (washing) and drainage (removal of infected material) of any involved areas. It may be necessary to remove an implant and leave it out for several weeks or months before it can be reinserted. When treated appropriately, infections normally resolve without significant long-term consequences, although some scar tissue can persist.

Surgical problems that may not be apparent until somewhat later include delayed healing, unfavorable scars, asymmetry, changes in sensation, persistent pain, and nerve injuries.

Not every undesirable consequence of surgery is legitimately considered a complication. The boundary between a normal consequence and a complication can be indistinct. For example, scarring is a normal part of all procedures. While narrow scars are preferable, a wide and/or uncomfortable scar is generally considered an unfavorable result rather than a complication. Plastic surgeons use careful planning, including the placement of incisions, and surgical technique to minimize potential scars. Fortunately, most incisions heal well. Exactly how wide or thick a scar has to be in order to be considered unfavorable has not been defined precisely. Scars normally fade quite acceptably (typically within several months, although it can take up to one or two years for a scar to mature completely), but there is no guarantee that they will do so. Different types of skin heal differently. In general, thicker skin heals less well (i.e., leaves worse scars) than thinner skin. Even on the same body, an incision on thin skin (like the upper eyelid) may heal well while one on thicker skin (like the upper back) may heal less favorably. Other factors contributing to the appearance of a scar include the orientation of the scar (vertical, horizontal, or oblique), the manner in which it was produced (a sharp laceration causes less tissue damage, and therefore produces a more favorable scar, than a jagged laceration, such as would be produced by a piece of glass), the way it was treated (i.e., sutured carefully, or left to heal on its own), and the amount of tension on the skin (greater tension produces a wider scar). Certain medical conditions (e.g., diabetes) and habits (e.g., tobacco use) can reduce blood flow and thereby increase the risk of complications.

The potential for complications exists with any surgical procedure and, unfortunately, it is not possible to guarantee complication-free surgery. On the other hand, prudent patient selection and care, skilled surgical techniques, anticipation, and early recognition and intervention make complications less likely to occur and, when they do, to minimize their impact.

CHAPTER 10

"Psychosurgery"

The actual meaning of "psychosurgery" is brain surgery that is done to treat psychic symptoms, i.e., symptoms of the mind. I use the term a little differently: to describe the magnified and beneficial effects that plastic surgery can have on people. Clearly, there are dramatic and stunning physical alterations that can be achieved. This is documented with photographs before and after surgery, and it is what initially draws most people to plastic surgery.

The effects on the whole person, however, often go far beyond the physical changes alone. The intensity of emotion associated with specific physical features can be impressive. Things easily ignored or accepted by some can be critically important to others. An example is one of my patients who underwent surgery to improve the appearance of her nose. This petite 19-year-old woman's nose had a large bump in the middle and a hook at the end and did not seem to fit with the rest of her face. As she awakened from her surgery, she suddenly burst into tears. Concerned that she was in pain or that there was some other problem, I asked her if she was okay. "I'm fine," she sobbed, "it's just that I've wanted this ever since I was thirteen." Another patient, a 31-year-old woman who had lost 100 pounds and then had a tummy tuck to remove the excess skin from her abdomen started crying during the unveiling of her new shape. "Do you realize," she said, "how long it's been since I had a nice stomach?"

Changing the appearance of one part of the body can have a generalized and lasting effect on the entire person. Increased self-confidence and a better self-image are widely mentioned as going along with an improved appearance. More than that is the happiness that plastic surgery can produce. People are happier in every way: about the way they look, about the way they feel, about the way clothes look on them, about the things people say to them, and about the way other people notice them. Six months after a 34-year-old mother of two had a tummy tuck, her husband remarked that she seemed so happy lately. She answered that she was; for the first time since "the kids," she was really comfortable with her body.

This is further illustrated by the experience of another of my patients, a business executive who wanted a liposuction. At 6' 0" tall and 140 pounds, she did not normally get sympathy from her friends. And yet, applying the same high standards to her body that she applied to her work, she was unhappy with her hips and outer thighs. She felt that they were disproportionate enough to keep her from wearing certain types of clothes, both for business (like suits with straight skirts) and for pleasure ("slinky" dresses, as she put it). It's not that she couldn't wear them — just that she didn't like the way she looked in them, and so she wouldn't wear them.

Several months after her liposuction, she gave a lecture to about 500 people. This was the fourth in a series, the first three having been before her procedure. She was wearing a suit that she had not been comfortable wearing previously. She looked great and she knew it; she also felt great. The overwhelming consensus was that this was by far her best speech yet. She later told me that the surgery made her look like the person she felt like inside. She also said that the increased confidence she had and the overall impression she'd made, a combination of substance and appearance, had been strengthened as a result of the liposuction. And enhanced that much further when she put on a slinky dress for the reception that followed....

It is expected that (a) there will be demonstrable physical improvement as a result of the plastic surgery and (b) patients will be pleased as a result of this improvement. As used here, the word "psychosurgery" represents the synergistic effect by which the whole is greater than the sum of its parts; essentially, that one plus one equals three. Patients' spirits are uplifted along with their bodies, and, for them, the gap between body and state of mind is bridged by plastic surgery.

CHAPTER 11

What If I Don't Like the Results?

Plastic surgeons go out of their way to prevent this situation from arising, and under ideal circumstances, it does not. Unfortunately, though, it can. In general, the elements of success in plastic surgery include a good candidate for the procedure in question, realistic expectations, and technically successful surgery.

To start with, not all things are possible for all people. As effective as plastic surgery procedures are, there are things they cannot accomplish. It is as important for patients to be told that what they want may not be possible as it is for patients to tell the doctors what they want. Once the patient's request has been stated, it is up to the surgeon to select the appropriate procedure(s). There may be more than one, but the wrong procedure, even if performed in a technically superb manner, will not produce the desired result.

With all procedures, realistic expectations, on the part of both patient and doctor, are important in leading to a success and preventing a disappointment. Most of the time expectations are realistic; one of the key functions of the consultation is to establish and ensure that. Despite everyone's best intentions and efforts, unrealistic expectations may persist. If the doctor feels that a patient's expectations are unrealistic despite appropriate explanation, he or she may decide not to perform the surgery. In extreme cases, psychiatric intervention may be the most appropriate treatment.

Ensuring that the patient and doctor are "on the same page" can be tricky. One of my first breast enlargements demonstrated this clearly. After the consultation the patient decided to have the surgery adding that, above all else, she did not want to be too big. She said that she wanted to be a full *B* cup, or possibly a small *C* at the absolute largest. I told her that I could do that, that proportions would be maintained, that it would look natural, etc. Over the next three weeks she called me almost daily to emphasize that she absolutely and definitely did not want to be too big. We discussed this in detail and I continued to reassure her. In my own mind, however, the size implant I intended to use went down a little bit each time I talked to her. (Implants come in volumes, not cup sizes — see Chapter 14). Eventually, I suggested that she bring in some pictures from a magazine showing the size she wanted to be. She arrived for her surgery clutching a handful of pages torn from various magazines. The smallest cup size displayed in the photos was a full *D*. She may not have realized what cup size she really wanted or she may have been embarrassed to admit it. Either way, a potential mix-up was averted only at the last minute, and the result was a happy patient.

Individual variations in healing (including scarring and qualities of the skin), recovery, and innumerable unknown factors may be responsible for otherwise predictable surgery producing unintended results. In addition, for any of a number of reasons, the surgeon may be largely responsible for an undesirable or unfavorable result.

Most problems can be solved, or at least minimized to the point where they are no longer an issue, although it may take another, revisional procedure to accomplish this. If it doesn't turn out the way the patient wants, potential correction or adjustment depends on what the problem is. This is different for different procedures. After liposuctions and breast reductions, for example, it is easier to take out a little more (at a later procedure) than to put some back. For breast enlargements, it is relatively easy to put in larger or smaller implants, or to remove them entirely, if that decision is made soon enough, i.e., within several months. Prominent scars can, in general, be improved with a scar revision (a procedure designed to improve the cosmetic and/or functional qualities of a scar). Often, several weeks or more should pass before anything else is done. For medical reasons it may not be safe or prudent to perform a second, non-emergent surgical procedure too soon after the first one.

It may also just be a question of waiting long enough. Swelling, which is a normal consequence of any surgery, can obscure the result. Waiting for some or most of the swelling to diminish often helps the patient to see that the surgery was, in fact, successful.

Finally, even if the result is not exactly what the patient thought it would be, it is usually a significant improvement over the preoperative appearance. Even when the expectations are realistic, it can be difficult for the patient to know precisely what he or she will look like after the surgery. As with other types of "renovations," sometimes it takes a while to get used to your new body.

Section 2
Breast Surgery

Breasts come in a tremendous range of shapes, sizes, and consistencies. Breasts are composed of skin, breast tissue, and fat. The relative proportions of these components vary, not only from individual to individual, but at different times of one person's life. The "ideal" breast is shaped essentially like a cone, with the widest part at the base (the portion that rests on the chest) and the peak at the nipple.

Breast tissue forms during puberty, developing from "buds" that are present at birth. While breasts are fully grown in most cases by the late teens or early twenties, their makeup and consistency continue to evolve throughout one's life. Even the size can fluctuate, depending on many factors. In young women, breasts are typically firm and relatively uplifted, and are composed primarily of glandular tissue with relatively little fat. With time, this changes. The breast tissue (i.e., the glands) is gradually replaced by fat, and the breasts begin or continue to sag. Pregnancy and weight gain or loss affect the breasts further. When sagging occurs as a result of pregnancy and breast-feeding, it is termed "involutional hypomastia," literally, small breasts caused by inward collapse of the breast tissue.

The age of onset and rate of progression of these processes vary considerably. Some women exhibit these changes in their teens or early twenties, with or without pregnancy. Others maintain youthful-appearing breasts much longer and despite pregnancy. As with many other features, heredity is an important determining factor.

There are essentially two types of procedures that can be done to breasts: augmentation (enlargement) and lift/reduction. Examination of the breasts will usually indicate which procedure (or combination) would be most effective in providing the desired result. As always, different surgeons may make different recommendations. Breast augmentation is accomplished by inserting an implant beneath the breast tissue, thereby enlarging the existing breast. Among the issues to consider are the type and size of the implant, the incision through which it is inserted, the precise location of the implant relative to the muscles of the chest, and whether or not a lift is required at the same time.

A lift/reduction is a procedure in which tissue is removed from the breast. The surgical techniques used for these two procedures are essentially identical. The type and amount of tissue removed determine whether it is called a lift or a reduction. When primarily skin, with or without a small amount of breast tissue, is removed, the procedure is called a lift, or mastopexy (literally "securing of the breast"). When more breast tissue is removed, it is called a breast reduction. Even in this case at least some skin is always removed. In both procedures the nipple position is normally raised. Exactly how much tissue has to be removed in order to qualify the procedure as a breast reduction is somewhat debatable. By one definition, if it is less than 300 grams (about 10 ounces) from each side, it is called a lift; if more, it is called a reduction.

Many different types of breast reduction procedures have been described and are in use. Various scar patterns are produced as a result of these procedures. Different surgeons may have preferences for specific procedures, and certain anatomical factors can influence the decision-making process. Even when a lift is combined with a breast enlargement, there are different techniques, and therefore scar patterns, to consider.

CHAPTER 12

Breast Enlargement (Augmentation)

Breast implant surgery is a procedure of instant gratification. It produces, almost without exception, an immediate and stunning transformation. The insertion of an implant beneath the breast tissue enlarges the breast and increases its projection, thereby increasing the cup size. The texture of the breast may also be changed, since breast implants often feel firmer than breast tissue.

In this surgery, an incision is made in the skin, an appropriate pocket or recipient site is created, and the implant is then inserted and placed in the correct position. The size of implant to be used can be determined before or during the surgery. There are many factors to consider with this surgery. There are different types of breast implants (saline-filled or silicone gel-filled), different coatings or shells of the implants (textured or smooth), different shapes of the implants themselves (round or anatomic), different anatomic locations in which the implant is placed (above or below the pectoral muscle), and different incisions through which they can be inserted (under the nipple, under the breast, and under the arm). Each of these options is discussed below; as always, there are advantages and disadvantages associated with each option. The surgery can be performed under intravenous sedation or general anesthesia. The particular operation chosen, with its varied options, is individualized, based on the preferences of the patient and the surgeon.

Breast enlargement is different conceptually from the other procedures described in this book. While the others are procedures of subtraction (i.e., skin, fat, and/or breast tissue are removed from the body), breast enlargement is a procedure of addition (i.e., something foreign — the implant — is added to the body). Most women who have had this procedure are extremely happy with their implants, but the ramifications of this central distinction constitute much of the discussion concerning breast enlargement.

CHAPTER 13

What Are Breast Implants?

Most breast implants currently in use in the United States are called saline implants. They are actually silicone bags that are filled with saline (salt water). The implants are inserted empty and are filled to a specific size once they are in position.

This was not always the case. The first solid implant was introduced in this country in 1962. Breast enlargement had been performed around the world for many years, but it had been accomplished by injecting any of a number of semi-liquid materials into the breast. For example, paraffin was used widely in Asia. Often there were disastrous results, as the paraffin could become infected, result in lumps and masses of scar tissue, and cause severe deformities of the skin and surrounding tissues. In the 1950s, implants made of a polyvinyl sponge called Ivalon were used. Although initial results were good, this material was ultimately abandoned. The porous nature of the sponge led to an unacceptable incidence of infection, and the implant was associated with a large number of complications, including hardness, irregularities, and asymmetry. In the 1960s, a rubber (silicone) was used in a new type of implant. Believed to be inert (i.e., non-reactive), it was formed into two slightly different versions: a firmer one used for the shell, or casing, and a looser one (gel), which was used to fill the implant. Silicone gel is an excellent match for the texture and consistency of normal, youthful breast tissue. The silicone implant revolutionized this surgery by providing a remarkably breast-like object that could be inserted to increase the size of the breast.

Capsules, or "Hard Breasts"

The first silicone implants were constructed with smooth outsides (shells), came prefilled to a specific size, and were placed directly underneath the breast tissue. The results were significantly better than what had been previously available. Eventually, however, one of the most common complications of breast implants first appeared: "capsules," also known as "hard breasts." A capsule is scar tissue that forms around an implant, and it represents the body's natural response to a foreign object. Capsules form in all cases of breast augmentation, but they usually remain soft and cannot be felt or distinguished from the breast tissue or implant. They can, however, become mildly or moderately firm; in extreme cases, they contract tightly into spherical, ball-like shapes. When this happens, the breasts become hard and round, may ride up higher on the chest, and can become painful. They also do not flatten out when the patient lies down.

Exact statistics concerning capsules are difficult to obtain. The subjectivity of the problem, women's happiness with their increased breast size even with capsules, and the private nature of plastic surgery have made accurate scientific studies hard to come by in this as well as other issues. In one review, however, the rate of capsules ranged from 10–50%. It has been noted that the incidence of capsules — whatever it is — only increases with time.

As breast capsules became more problematic, two major modifications were developed in an attempt to prevent them. Neither approach guaranteed that a capsule would not form, but both improved the odds. One alteration was to place them in a deeper anatomic location. Instead of placing them directly under the breast tissue, surgeons started inserting them underneath, (i.e., behind or below), the pectoral muscle, which is the main chest muscle. Often referred to as "the pecs," these muscles are relatively thin in an average woman. They provide a cover for the implant (which can be beneficial, particularly with certain types of implants), and there are certain advantages, from a cosmetic standpoint, to having the implants beneath the muscle (termed submuscular) — these are discussed more fully below. This is particularly true for thin patients. From a functional standpoint, the constant motion of the muscle, with its flexing action on the implant, apparently inhibits the formation of a clinically troublesome capsule. While capsules can form with submuscular implants, they appear to do so less commonly. In an extension of this concept, many surgeons advise their patients to massage and manipulate their implants daily, attempting to duplicate the natural actions of the pectoral muscles. Despite widespread advocacy of this massage, the scientific basis for making these recommendations has not been definitively established. The treatment of capsules is discussed in Chapters 15 and 18.

Textured or Smooth?

Another approach in the fight against capsules was to redesign the implant itself. It was determined that, compared with a smooth-shelled implant placed above the muscle, an irregular and rough shell (or casing) decreased the likelihood that the capsule would contract into a spherical shape. This rough shell is now referred to as textured, as opposed to smooth. Silicone gel implants constructed in this fashion included those made entirely of silicone and those that had a polyurethane foam coating attached to the silicone shell. Both textured and smooth saline implants are available and are used widely. Because of the way it is manufactured, the shell of a textured saline implant is a little thicker than that of a smooth implant. The consequences of these structural differences are discussed in further detail on the following pages.

The Silicone Gel Controversy

The silicone breast implant controversy of the early 1990s made the implant unavailable to the American public in most cases, thereby reducing the options for the average breast implant candidate. There have been a number of medical and surgical problems in patients who have silicone gel breast implants. Both local and systemic complications have been reported. The local mechanical problems, such as capsular contractures, infections, silicone bleed (ooze), ruptures, and resultant scar tissue, appear to be consequences of the implants themselves. The systemic medical problems that have been reported, such as autoimmune reactions or diseases (also referred to as collagen-vascular diseases), weakness, etc., are linked more tenuously. The simultaneous presence of two conditions does not automatically confer cause and effect. The scientific link between silicone gel breast implants and the problems in the patients who received them is debatable and is the subject of ongoing controversy. The most recent scientific reviews, however, conclude that there is no link between these implants and an increased risk of either autoimmune diseases or cancer.[8,9] Furthermore, medical grade silicone, which is related to silicone gel, is used in a wide range of products, including pharmaceuticals, cosmetics, over-the-counter preparations, and in food processing. Adults and children regularly inhale, absorb, and are otherwise exposed to this compound. Regardless, health concerns related to the use of silicone gel implants have eliminated their use from consideration for most prospective patients in the United States. They continue to be widely available in other countries around the world.

Silicone gel breast implants are, however, still available in this country in a limited number of circumstances. Several hundred plastic surgeons are participating in investigative studies of these implants, which can be used in breast reconstruction patients (i.e., after mastectomies for breast cancer) and when, for any number of reasons (see below), saline implants are inadequate. Patients who agree to enter these investigations must sign an extensive consent form and

[8] Angell, M. Evaluating the health risks of breast implants: the interplay of medical science, the law and public opinion. *The New England Journal of Medicine.* 334:1513, 1996. This topic is explored more fully in Dr. Angell's book, *Science on Trial*, New York, W. W. Norton & Company, 1997.

[9] Brinton, I. Breast implants and cancer. *J. Natl. Cancer Inst.* 89:1341, 1997

undergo a series of medical assessments, both before and after their procedures. Criteria for inclusion in the studies include postmastectomy reconstruction, severe deformities (traumatic or congenital), replacements for patients who already have the gel implants, and saline implant failure or unsuitability. The latter includes insufficient breast tissue or skin and waviness or rippling of the implants. Information derived from the studies is being used to assess the implants and their suitability for continued use.

One possibly beneficial consequence of the silicone controversy is a wider understanding that breast implants, in general, may not be permanent. A certain percentage of women who undergo this procedure may need replacement or revisions of some kind. This first became apparent in silicone gel cases, but is true for saline implants as well.

New breast implants are currently under development, including some that have an improved consistency (when compared with saline implants) and are more radiolucent (i.e., X-rays pass through them better), thereby increasing the effectiveness of mammograms. This would be a significant advantage since X-rays are largely blocked by both silicone and saline implants, which makes it harder to assess breast tissue accurately with mammograms. Extensive testing is required before any new implant becomes available. That process takes time and resources on the part of the manufacturers, and liability concerns are significant. For these reasons, among others, developing a new implant is an enormous undertaking.[10]

Saline Implants

The first major alternative to the silicone gel implant was an inflatable implant, which was introduced in 1965. Filled with saline (salt water), which is a natural component of the

[10] For example, the Trilucent® implant (a silicone shell filled with triglycerides derived from peanut oil, whose major advantage was better visualization of breast tissue on mammograms) was withdrawn from clinical trials pending reports of several problems, leaving its future in doubt.

body, the shell of this implant is constructed of silicone but is thicker than the shell of the silicone gel implant. This is because of differences between silicone gel, which holds its shape relatively well (like gelatin), and saline, which like water is completely dependent on its "container" to give it any shape. A cup of silicone gel placed on a table would, more or less, hold its shape while a cup of saline poured on a table would run right off. Saline implants, therefore, require a thicker shell than silicone gel implants; this makes them feel somewhat firmer than gel implants.

Saline implants have had their proponents as long as they've been available. Since saline is a naturally occurring substance, it is theoretically less of a medical problem than silicone gel. Additionally, because the implants are inserted empty and filled with saline once they're in place, they can be inserted through smaller incisions than would be required for prefilled implants of the same size.

Both textured and smooth saline implants are used widely. The choice of implants depends on the relative importance that is placed on the advantages and disadvantages of each type. The use of textured implants appears to lower the incidence of capsule formation when compared with smooth-walled implants. There are several features that are unique to textured implants. Because a textured implant grabs the tissue, an implant will remain, to a large extent, wherever it is placed. This is an advantage when positioning the implant. On the other hand, the shell of the textured implant is a little thicker than that of the smooth implant. The combination of texturing and a thicker shell is associated with a disadvantage that can occur with this implant: rippling. As the tissue heals around the implant, the implant may fold slightly in one or more areas. This can occur with smooth implants also, but seems to be more common with textured implants. Rippling, when present, can occur to varying degrees. Often it can be felt, particularly around the lower and outer edges of the implant, and in extreme cases the ripples may be visible through the skin.

Many surgeons use smooth implants, particularly for placement behind the muscle. The thinner shell of the smooth implant is an advantage because it may be less noticeable to the touch than the thicker shell of the textured implant. From a technical standpoint, it is a little easier for the surgeon to work with in one sense, but harder in another. Because of the thinner and smoother shell, it folds into a smaller shape and can be inserted more easily through a small incision and guided into whatever position is desired. On the other hand, because it is smooth and a little slippery, it may slide down to the lowermost edge (or sometimes up to the upper, outer part) of the pocket, or space, that has been created for it. The pockets, therefore, must be created with absolute precision. A smooth implant is less forgiving of any asymmetry in the creation of the pockets than a textured implant is.

Finally, capsules are the most troublesome consequences of saline breast implants. Although the evidence is not absolute, many surgeons feel that smooth implants are more likely to develop capsules than textured, and it is this reasoning that often persuades them to recommend textured implants. It may take a while (months or years) for the capsules to form, and exercises (massage, displacement, etc.) may help delay or prevent the scarring, but there is supporting evidence[11] that smooth implants are eventually associated with a higher rate of capsular contracture than are textured implants.

Round or Anatomic?

Implants also come in two general shapes: round and anatomic. A round implant is round when viewed from the front (i.e., when viewed from the top if the implant is lying on a table); the diameters of both its height and its width are the same. An anatomic implant is slightly oval when viewed from the front, and it protrudes in a low, conical fashion when viewed from the side. Relatively more of its volume is in the lower portion of the implant. In this manner, the anatomic implant more closely duplicates the shape of a natural breast

---

[11] Among others, Asplund, O. Textured or smooth implants for submuscular breast augmentation: a controlled study. *Plast. Reconstr. Surg.* 97:1200, 1996.

than a round implant. Developed initially for use in breast reconstruction (after mastectomy), it is now used in cosmetic procedures also. One disadvantage of the anatomic implant is that it is somewhat more difficult to orient correctly since even a slight rotation will produce asymmetry. Round implants, for this reason, are a little easier to place. Additionally, the superior (upper) fullness of the round implant (i.e., as much volume is in the upper half as in the lower half), is considered desirable by many women. That superior fullness contributes to more prominent cleavage and a "lifted" look.

Other types of implants have been introduced since the 1960s, but most did not gain wide acceptance and have not lasted. One implant of note was a double-lumen or chambered implant. This implant had two compartments: one filled with silicone and one filled with saline. Depending on the particular make of the implant, either filling (silicone or saline) was on the inside with the other surrounding it. Some surgeons reported better results with this type of implant than with other types.

Above or Below the Muscle?

An important consideration is where, with respect to the chest muscles, the implant will be placed. The main chest muscles are the pectorals (the "pecs"), and the implant can be placed in one of two possible locations: (1) directly under the breast (above the muscle or subparenchymal) or (2) deep to the muscle (below the muscle or submuscular). (See Figure 1). As always, there are advantages and disadvantages with each. Some surgeons use one location all or most of the time; others vary it depending on many factors. Even when the implant is under the muscle, it is not entirely under the muscle. The outer, lower third of the implant, or more (depending on the size of the implant), may be under the skin and breast tissue, since the pectoral muscle (actually the pectoralis major — there are two other, smaller pectoral muscles) does not extend over the entire position of the implant. Some surgeons

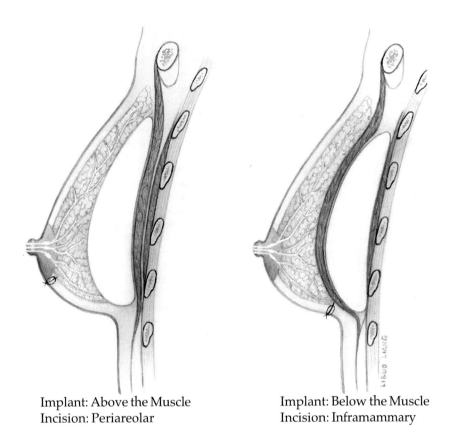

Implant: Above the Muscle
Incision: Periareolar

Implant: Below the Muscle
Incision: Inframammary

Figure 1. Breast Implants: Above / Below the Muscle

incorporate portions of other nearby muscles so that the implant is completely submuscular.

There are specific advantages of subpectoral implants. Placing the implant beneath the pectoral muscle is particularly beneficial for patients who are very thin. When there is inadequate skin and breast tissue, an implant placed on top of the muscle may be too easily felt and seen. Placing it beneath the muscle diminishes this problem. A patient may have more of a sense that the implant is a part of her, rather than being as exposed, to both sight and touch, as an implant directly under the breast would be. Another advantage is the decreased likelihood of capsule formation. The constant motion of the pectoral muscle may explain the finding that capsules are less common with submuscular breast implants. Yet another advantage of implants in this location is that the muscle helps to hold and support the implant. Over time, this internal "bra" may help prevent sagging more than if the skin alone has to support the implants.

Aside from any aesthetic considerations, there are several medical advantages to having the implants below the muscle rather than on top of it. Physicians typically find that a breast is more easily examined and possible masses are more easily assessed, both manually and radiographically, when the implant is a little further away from the breast tissue. Even the thickness of the muscle (which in the average, non-bodybuilder woman is less than half an inch) over the implant provides an effective landmark and point of differentiation for the examiner. Similarly, a mammogram (an X-ray of the breast) can better assess and identify the exact location and characteristics of any suspicious lesions, including both those that can be felt and those that are visible only on the mammogram. Despite some controversy, there is no proven increase in the risk of cancer associated with any breast implants. However, the cornerstone of the treatment of breast cancer remains early detection, and anything that facilitates that is potentially to the patient's advantage.

While advantageous in many ways, placing the implants under the muscle is, in a sense, a more unnatural position. In both cases, the skin has to stretch to make room for the implant. In the submuscular position, the muscle has to stretch, too. The larger the implant, the greater the accommodation that will be required by the muscle. This process starts during the surgery itself, but may take several weeks to complete. In addition, the implants may feel slightly firmer, particularly right after the surgery, than if they are placed on top of the muscle. Over the next several weeks and months they soften and assume a more natural shape and look.

Bodybuilders (as well as aerobic instructors, racket sports athletes, etc.) often decide to have their implants placed on top of the muscle. The basis for this actually stems from the use of smooth-walled implants. When these implants are placed under the muscle and the muscles are flexed (contracted), the implants may jump to the side. The implants return to their position as soon as the muscle relaxes; while not uncomfortable, the movement of the implant can be unsightly. Though more common with smooth-walled implants, this can also occur with textured implants. This concern leads these women to have their implants placed on top of the muscle. This option, however, is not without disadvantages of its own. These patients tend to have very little body fat. Their breasts have all but disappeared as a result of their extreme training and dieting. With implants on top of the muscle, one sees the skin stretched tightly over the implants; the implants can look as though they were literally "stuck onto" the chest. Despite this, many patients opt for this location to prevent any movement of the implant when the pectoral muscles are flexed.

Patients with adequate skin and breast tissue may have good results with implants on top of the muscle. One advantage of placing the implant above the muscle is that the location is somewhat more natural. If the skin of the breasts is stretched and there is a small to moderate amount of sagging, an implant above the muscle may fill this space out nicely. Patients who have enough breast tissue to cover the implant are more likely to do well with the implant in this location, but even in this case, the implant can be felt more easily than if it is below the muscle. Many surgeons believe that implants placed on top of the muscle will be more likely to develop one or more problems with time. When placed in this position the rippling that may develop with textured implants is more likely to be noticeable, the implants may be more likely to sag, and smooth implants may be more likely to develop capsules. Since capsule formation is the biggest problem with saline implants, preventing them is the overriding concern.

In the midst of the confusion surrounding the choices of implant and location, surgeons have to decide what they prefer to use and under what circumstances. Some surgeons vary the implant style and/or location depending on the situation; others always (or nearly so) use the same implant type and location. With time, trends, even if short-term, become apparent. It appears that plastic surgeons increasingly prefer smooth implants as they gain experience in the post–silicone gel era. One potential concern is whether this trend represents a short-term benefit; it may be that the rippling and stiffness that are more common with textured implants are simply becoming apparent sooner than capsules, which represent the major concern with smooth implants.

Despite all the choices available, the most important factor in predicting the result of a breast enlargement may be the amount of breast tissue present before the surgery. The more breast tissue, the better the result is likely to be, regardless of which type of implant is used. This is because having relatively more breast tissue provides a cover and helps to camouflage any imperfections related to the implant itself. The larger the implant relative to the existing breast tissue, the more likely the implant will be noticeable. At its extreme, a large implant coupled with a very small breast, even if placed in the subpectoral position, may sag eventually to the point where it is mostly subglandular and even subcutaneous, i.e., directly under the skin, leaving any resulting imperfections that much more evident. Clearly, however, this is somewhat unavoidable. Most of these patients don't have a lot of breast tissue to begin with; if they did, they wouldn't be having this surgery.

Which Incision?

Another issue is the incision through which the implant is inserted. There are three incisions used most commonly and excellent results can be achieved with all three (See Figure 2). They are the periareolar (around the areola, which is the dark area around the nipple), inframammary (under or beneath the breast), and axillary (under the arm, within the armpit). A fourth incision (umbilical, or through the belly button), is used only rarely. As before, surgeon and/or patient preference determine which of the incisions is used; the choice of incision does not guarantee a specific result. Any type of implant (textured or smooth, round or anatomic) can be inserted through any of the three main incisions and placed into either position (above or below the muscle).

The patient's major concerns tend to be how well hidden each one is and what impact each may have on nipple and breast sensation.

The first depends somewhat on how "hidden" is defined. As with all scars, there is tremendous variation from person to person as well as in different areas on the same person. All scars are permanent, but the eventual appearance of a scar depends on many factors, including where on the body and in what orientation it is, how the scar was produced, how much tension the scar is under, and the technique by which it was repaired. Scars in all three locations range from barely discernible to obvious. With one's clothes off and the lights on, a well-healed axillary incision is probably the most difficult to identify. A few years ago, before it was in wide usage, the axillary incision was an even better choice in terms of camouflage than it is today. The periareolar and inframamma-

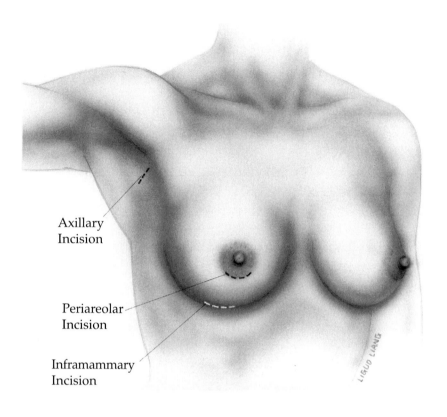

Axillary
Incision

Periareolar
Incision

Inframammary
Incision

Figure 2.   Breast Implant Incisions

ry incisions were better known; having relatively large breasts and no visible scars on the breast was a novelty. Now, with axillary incisions used more often, the fact that they may be visible even when women wear something sleeveless — such as a bathing suit, exercise outfit, or evening gown — can be a disadvantage. If the healing is less than optimal, the scar or an indentation in the axilla can be noticeable in many different situations. In a sense, the periareolar incision may be the most hidden. It is completely hidden in any bathing suit top, bra, or any clothing and is visible, if at all, only when one's top is off — as are all the incisions. Proponents of the inframammary incision cite that it is hidden from view by the natural hang of the breast when the patient is standing. It may, however, be more noticeable if the patient is lying down, and a bathing suit or similar top may ride up, exposing the scar.

Patients are also concerned about the effect the surgery and the incision will have on the sensation of the breast and, in particular, the nipple. Many claims have been made about the impact that implant size, location, and choice of incision have on sensation, but there is relatively little documentation. One study designed to compare the incisions concluded that the most important determining factor in preserving nipple sensation was the size of the implant, rather than the choice of incision.[12] The larger the implant, the greater the possibility that sensation would be impaired. This makes sense inherently, as a larger implant requires that a larger pocket be created, which disrupts more of the nerve fibers that supply the skin. This study considered only implants placed on top of the muscle. There is certainly some potential loss of sensation with breast enlargement surgery. In general, much of this is temporary, but it can take up to six months for most — and two years for all — of the sensation to return. My experience is that sensation is preserved at least as well, if not better, with implants placed below the muscle than above it, and that the incision does not per se guarantee or preclude any result. Many women have reported that their sensation

---

[12] Courtiss, E. Breast sensation before and after plastic surgery. *Plast. Reconstr. Surg.* 58:1, 1976.

was enhanced by this surgery. While a comprehensive, scientifically valid study has not been published, one recent report concluded that postoperative sensation was not related either to the implant location (above or below the muscle) or the incision used.[13]

There are additional considerations. Compared with the other two incisions, the axillary incision is situated further away from where the implants are placed. For that reason, it is technically more difficult to achieve correct placement of the implants. After the implants are inserted during the surgery, the patient is raised into a sitting position on the Operating Room table, and the position of one or both of the implants must often be adjusted. It is tricky enough to do this under normal circumstances, since swelling, small amounts of bleeding and/or any local anesthesia injected may make this determination difficult. Because of the greater distance, it is that much more difficult to do this from the axillary position. Additionally, if there is excessive bleeding during the surgery, one of the other two incisions must often be made in order to achieve control. Smooth implants, because of their ability to slide easily, are often preferred with the axillary incision.

The umbilical incision became an option after the endoscope was introduced into plastic surgery. An endoscope is a lighted, optical tube through which one can see inside the body. Using incisions in and around the umbilicus (belly button), a tunnel is created from that area to each breast. The implant is inserted through the umbilicus and put into position beneath each breast. For mechanical reasons, however, it is necessary to use a smooth implant (a textured implant will not slide well enough within the endoscope) and to place it on top of the muscle (it is too difficult to place the implant beneath the muscle from that far away). The combination of smooth implants on top of the muscle is often considered undesirable, as it may lead to an increased risk of capsular contracture. Concern has been raised that the tracks of the endoscope (i.e., the V-shaped pattern extending from

---

[13] Young, V. L. Nipple-areolar sensibility following augmentation mammaplasty. Presented at ASAPS Meeting, New York, May 1997.

the umbilicus to each breast) may ultimately become visible. For these reasons, as well as the technical difficulty in accurately placing the implants, there has been a relatively high rate of dissatisfaction with this approach.

Finally, a note on the immediate postoperative appearance of breast implants. It may take a while (several weeks or months) before the final results of this surgery can be appreciated. Since swelling is typically maximized at 2–3 days after the surgery, assessment at this point may give a slightly false impression. Patients may be somewhat larger in the first few days after surgery than they will be ultimately. Also, the shape of the breast may be flattened and broad initially, particularly with submuscular implants. With time the skin and breast tissue (and muscle, if the implants have been placed under it) relax and adapt to the contour of the implant, resulting in a much more natural shape and feel.

CHAPTER 14

Choosing the Right Size Implant

Choosing the right size breast implant can be tricky. The following is a method of determining which size saline implant will produce the desired result. Since the implant is placed under the skin and breast tissue, and possibly under the muscle, there is no way to show exactly what it will be like. This system, however, has been effective in simulating the result. It is designed for women who do not currently have breast implants. Taking measurements in the presence of implants, particularly if there are capsules, is more complicated.

Breast shapes and sizes vary tremendously. Cup sizes are designed to be independent of body type — a C cup is supposed to be the same from woman to woman, regardless of her height and weight. Implants, however, need to be individualized. An implant that provides a full breast on a woman with a narrow ribcage may be lost on a woman with a wider ribcage, regardless of the preoperative cup size. Further complicating implant selection is the fact that some women like their bra to fit snugly, and others loosely.

Saline implants do not come in cup sizes. Instead, they come in a variety of sizes which are measured in cc (cubic centimeters, or milliliters). There are 30 cc in an ounce and 1000 cc in a liter (which is about a quart). Since a liter of saline weighs a little over two pounds, a 250 cc saline implant weighs just over half a pound. Each implant is designed to be filled to a specific volume.

In order to do this test, you should first buy a bra of the size you want to be (after doing this you may want a different size; in that case, buy a new bra and start the process again). Then, get 4 or 5 plastic baggies with twisties (some people prefer using balloons), a marker, and one or two quarts of warm water. Do not use Ziploc®-type bags and make sure the water is not too hot or too cold — the reasons will become evident! Fill the baggies, two at a time, with specific amounts of water — 8 ounces, 10 ounces, etc. These volumes correspond to particular implants, and the amounts you should use are suggested by the surgeon based on the consultation. Take the filled baggie, squeeze out as much excess air as possible, and close it with a twistie. Dry the outside of the baggie, mark the size, and then put it inside your bra. Try to flatten it out so that it fills the cup as widely as possible (i.e., don't let it stay balled up or too rounded). Another way to do this is to use sample implants which may be available in the doctor's office.

This approximates the way the implant will fill the bra. Of course, the baggie is on top of the skin while the actual implant is compressed beneath the skin, breast tissue, and possibly, the muscle. It is sometimes necessary to use one size larger implant than would be indicated by this test in order to achieve the desired result, particularly with submuscular placement. Nevertheless, this gives an idea of what the post-operative result will look like and what it will feel like to carry some extra weight on your chest.

When the patient already has implants, with or without capsules, the measurements become more complicated. This system can still be used, but the surgeon must take many more factors into account when deciding which implant to use.

CHAPTER 15

Surgery to Redo Breast Implants

There are a number of reasons why a woman who currently has breast implants may want or need to change them. First, assuming there are no other problems with them, a woman may not like the size. It is simpler to go to a larger size than to go to a smaller size; the reasons for this are discussed below. Tightness of the breast skin and tissue may have limited the size of implant that could be inserted at the initial procedure. With time, however, the tissues stretch, allowing the insertion of a larger implant at a later procedure. Larger implants can be put in the same location (i.e., above or below the muscle) or in a different one. Either way, it is necessary to increase the size of the pocket, or space, for the implant.

It is a little more complicated if a woman wants her breasts made smaller. While it is relatively simple to remove larger implants and replace them with smaller ones, the problems are the skin and the size of the pocket. Over time, the skin of the breast (and if applicable the pectoral muscle) stretches to accommodate the breast implant. This helps explain why it takes several months to see the final result after the surgery. The reverse, unfortunately, is not necessarily true. As is evidenced routinely (for example, the stomach after a pregnancy), skin may not have adequate elasticity and the ability to tighten up when the larger item underneath it is removed. If one is going from a larger to a smaller implant, it may be necessary to perform a breast lift and/or raise the lower edge of the implant (a smaller implant in the same pocket may slide down and be too low — see below). A lift can be done at the same time or at a later date. Skin can and does contract to a certain extent, and muscle usually contracts adequately. For that reason, and because the lift procedures leave more scarring than an enlargement or replacement procedure alone, if there is a question as to whether or not one needs a lift, it is often more prudent to delay the decision. Breast lifts following implant replacement can often be performed under local anesthesia with light sedation and have a milder recovery than the implant portion of the procedure. It is easier to add the lift procedure later than it is to take away the scars if one didn't really need it.

Another reason to undergo the removal and replacement of breast implants is if they are in the wrong position (too high, too low, etc.). Implants may have shifted with time, or they may have been placed incorrectly during the initial procedure. Gravity constantly works to drag the breasts (and everything else!) down into a lower position, and surgery may be required to raise them.

As always, some things are easier to correct than others. It is easier to lower implants than to raise them. This is because lowering the implant involves simply extending the bottom edge of the pocket, repositioning the implant, and allowing gravity to keep it in the new location. If a small implant is inserted into the pocket previously occupied by a large implant, it may slide down to the lower edge of the pocket, leaving it too low in relation to the breast. This is essentially what has already occurred if an implant is too low. In each case, the position of the implant must be raised. The new, raised lower edge of the pocket is created by inserting a series of stitches (sutures) that block the implant from redescending. From a technical standpoint, this can be somewhat tricky. Scar tissue forms with time to help maintain the new position, but it is easier to work with gravity than against it. Moving the implant from side to side involves both enlarging the pocket on one side (inner or outer) and, often, making it smaller on the other.

A third reason to undergo breast implant replacement surgery is if there is a mechanical problem with the existing implant. For example, implants may have developed hard or painful capsules. These capsules can be removed and a new implant placed in the same or a different location, a textured implant may be used to replace a smooth one, or both approaches can be used. Capsules can be difficult to eradicate permanently as they can reform after having been removed. Additionally, breast implants can rupture or deflate, often as a result of an injury. Technical advances in the design and manufacture of implants have made these complications rare, but if they do occur the implants need to be replaced. Reoperation for any reason carries the same risks as the previous procedure(s).

Patients with silicone gel breast implants, with or without capsules, sometimes want to have them removed. Despite significant controversy and ongoing litigation, the latest evidence indicates that they do not cause medical problems. Nevertheless, and even with what would otherwise be considered excellent results, some women opt to have the implants removed. Most of the time they are replaced with saline implants. Sometimes, they are removed and not replaced; in this case, a breast lift is often advisable.

Ironically, it can go the other way, too. In this country, women can get silicone implants if they have a problem with their saline implants. Patients who could not have received silicone implants when they didn't have any implants at all may become eligible if, after getting saline implants at their first operation, they have enough of an unfavorable result to be included in the ongoing investigation. Rippling and excess visibility of the implants are among the problems that may qualify a patient for inclusion in the silicone implant studies (see "The Silicone Gel Controversy").

Finally, some patients who had silicone implants removed and replaced with saline implants have become dissatisfied with their new implants. Rippling and/or the overall feel of the implant may contribute to this dissatisfaction. This has led to renewed interest in any alternatives, including silicone. Some women who went from silicone to saline go back to silicone again. Aesthetically, silicone gel implants can produce remarkably good results. Some of the best results in breast enlargement surgery have been with silicone gel implants; unfortunately, so have some of the worst. Nevertheless, appreciation of the superior results possible with silicone gel has made the return of this implant, once considered unimaginable, a possibility — however unlikely.

CHAPTER 16

Enlargement with a Lift

Depending on the anatomy, it may be advisable to perform a lift in combination with a breast enlargement. Breast lifts are discussed in further detail below, along with breast reductions. There are actually many different procedures within the category termed "lifts." A breast lift accomplishes two things: It lifts the nipple into a higher position and it tightens the skin. Depending on the degree of sagging, it may be beneficial to add a lift to the enlargement. Sagging is associated with a loss of superior fullness of the breasts; i.e., the upper half of the breast is flat and much of the existing breast tissue is in the lower half and/or below the nipple. When there is little or no sagging, excellent results are normally achieved by inserting an implant alone; a lift is not required under these circumstances. If there is moderate to severe sagging, then an implant alone is normally not enough to produce the desired result. In this case, excess breast skin must be removed, in addition to inserting the implants. Finally, if existing breast implants are being replaced with smaller implants or removed altogether, a lift may be indicated, since the skin contracture and/or sagging that can otherwise occur in these cases may be undesirable. Even then, the decision to undergo the lift portion of the procedure can be delayed; some women may choose not to have it done at all.

There are other procedures that can accomplish breast enlargement with a lift, but they are generally reserved for breast reconstruction patients, i.e., patients who have had mastectomies for the treatment of breast cancer. For example, there is a way to reconstruct a breast by transferring one's own tissue from the abdomen to the chest. This procedure (called a "TRAM Flap") has been done in cases of severe disfigurement after breast implant surgery, particularly from silicone gel breast implants. An added benefit is that, in removing the abdominal tissue, a tummy tuck is performed. There are other procedures similar to this. One type transfers muscle (with or without skin) from the back to the breast, although an implant is generally required in this case in order to produce enough bulk. Another, using microsurgery, transfers tissue from the buttock region to the breast. In general, procedures of this scope are too involved, in terms of both the surgery and the recovery, for an otherwise healthy woman who wishes cosmetic improvement of her breasts.

CHAPTER 17

Tuberous Breasts

A tuberous breast is a variant of breast shape. As noted previously, the "ideal breast" is shaped like a cone with the widest part at the base (the portion that rests on the pectoral muscle). In tuberous breasts, the base of the breast is too tight for the remainder of the breast. When the base is narrowed or constricted, the breast tissue is forced forward into the areola. The breasts appear small and misshapen — "tube-like." Correction of this anatomical variant has two components. First, the undersurface of the base is released by making, from the inside, a radial (starburst) pattern of incisions or cuts on the base of the breast. This allows the breast to spread open and lie flat. Next, breast implants are inserted, either above or below the muscle. Aside from enlarging the breasts, the implants are needed to maintain the correction produced by the radial cuts, which would otherwise collapse and allow the tubular arrangement to form again. This combination of maneuvers is effective in correcting the deformity (see Patient # 12).

CHAPTER 18

Complications of Breast Implants

Complications of this surgery, as with others, fit into two general categories: those that appear early (within approximately the first two weeks after surgery), and those that appear late. Early complications are typically due to the surgery itself and are more urgent than late ones, which are commonly due to problems with the implant. A number of temporary conditions can occur, such as burning, itching, and a feeling of tightness; these are not generally considered complications. More complete disclosure statements are provided by the implant manufacturers.

The most significant early complication is excessive bleeding. The hallmark of excessive bleeding after breast enlargement is when one breast is significantly larger and more painful than the other in the first few hours or days after surgery; lesser degrees of asymmetry are common. It does not usually appear outside that time frame, although it can. Excessive bleeding may necessitate reoperation with removal of the blood and, if necessary, the implant, as well as renewed attempts at controlling the bleeding. In most cases, the implant can be reinserted at the same time; rarely (depending on the extent of the bleeding) it cannot. In that case, it can usually be inserted during a second procedure several weeks later. The delay may be necessary to ensure that the bleeding will not restart and that enough of the resultant swelling, which may cause a fluid buildup around the implant, can subside.

Infection is another potential complication. An infection may not become apparent until several days, weeks, or even months after the surgery. It typically appears as pain, swelling, and redness of one breast and may be associated with fever, chills, sweats, and other generalized signs of infection. Treatment consists of reoperation with the removal of any blood and/or infected material as well as the implant, and renewed or stronger antibiotics. It is not generally considered prudent to reinsert an implant during an active infection, as the presence of a foreign body (i.e., the implant) can prolong and worsen the course of the infection. The implant can be replaced after the infection has subsided completely, a process that may take several weeks or months. Understandably, this interim period, with an implant in only one side (the side that did not get infected), is unpleasant.

Once the first few weeks have passed, the likelihood of either of these problems appearing diminishes rapidly. Other problems, however, can become apparent; among these is capsules, or hard breasts. As noted above, this is part of the body's natural reaction to having a foreign substance within it. It can occur to varying degrees. When mild to moderate, there is relatively little that can be done. Up until a few years ago, capsules were treated by being "popped"; under light sedation, the surgeon used his or her hands literally to break the capsule. This procedure has been largely abandoned because the risk of implant rupture or capsular distortion outweighs the potential benefits of breaking the capsule. (There was also a relatively high incidence of injuries to the surgeon's hands!) For more severe cases, treatment consists of removal of the implant and, usually, replacement with another implant (the same or a different type), changing the position of the implant (with respect to the pectoral muscle), releasing and/or removing the scar tissue, or a combination of the above. Even this is not always successful. If there is excessive sagging of the skin, a lift can be performed to tighten the skin, usually elevating the nipple at the same time.

Other potential problems include changes in sensation and nipple reactivity (although these tend to be, if anything, heightened and improved by this surgery), leakage/deflation, fluid accumulation around the implant, and prolonged discomfort, particularly during certain movements. Decreased sensation is often temporary and may correspond to the size of implant relative to the chest size rather than to any particular incision, technique, or style of implant. Some degree of discomfort in the early postoperative period is to be expected. This is particularly true when the implants are placed in the subpectoral position. The discomfort tends to be minimal when the patient is not moving, but worse with movement and at night. Most of the problems associated with breast implants tend to resolve with time, which is fortunate: aside from removing the implants, there is often relatively little that can be done if the problems persist. In some cases, even removing the implants does not eliminate all the symptoms.

Finally, breast implant surgery does not appear to affect lactation, i.e., the breast's ability to produce milk. This is because the implants are placed either directly beneath the breast tissue, or even deeper — beneath the muscle that is under the breast. Patients with implants are routinely able to breast feed as well as women without implants can.

CHAPTER 19

Are My Implants Okay?

Women who have breast implants may, at some point in their lives, become concerned that something is wrong with their implants. Many problems, including hard capsules and deflation, are readily apparent; others, such as leakage, may not be. Despite the relative lack of scientific evidence supporting the hazards of silicone gel implants, most medical concerns, when present, are related to these implants. Saline-filled implants are of less concern for at least two reasons. First, the saline itself is not considered medically harmful. Saline (salt water) is similar to existing body fluids. If the implants leak, the saline is rapidly absorbed into the body where it appears to have no further consequences. Secondly, if saline implants leak or deflate, the problem usually becomes obvious quite rapidly as one side becomes much smaller or flattens completely.

Under ideal circumstances there would be a simple, accurate and inexpensive way to assess breast implants. At present, however, there isn't. Instead, there are two general ways of assessing breast implants: physical exams and non-invasive tests (i.e., X-rays and related examinations). Blood tests have not proven to be useful.

First and foremost is the physical exam. A change in the appearance or consistency of the breasts and/or breast implants may be an indication of a mechanical problem. It is not uncommon for breasts and implants to feel different at various points of the menstrual cycle, or in relation to one's hormonal or fluid status. Women often report that their breasts and implants, while generally soft, feel firmer at times. Nevertheless, such changes can also be associated with problems with the implants. If a breast becomes increasingly firm or changes size over a period of months and does not return to its normal, softer state, it may mean that a troublesome capsule is forming. Another indication is if portions of the implant become distorted (i.e., protrude in one or more directions, or develop bulges).

The next step is generally one or more non-invasive diagnostic tests, also called imaging. These include mammograms, sonograms (ultrasounds), CT Scans, and MRIs. All are performed under the supervision of radiologists, some of whom specialize in breast and breast implant imaging. Mammograms and sonograms may also be performed at gynecologists' and other doctors' offices. Diagnostic tests are not 100% accurate. Sometimes they miss things that are there (false negative results), and sometimes they see things that aren't really there (false positives).

Mammograms are standard X-rays of the breasts. The breast is compressed between two plates, and different views are taken. Women who have implants should make it known to the radiology technician so that particular caution can be used during the mammography; even then, they may be uncomfortable during this test. Implants placed under the muscle interfere less with mammography than those that are on top of the muscle. Mammograms are not as useful in assessing breast implants as one might think. Both silicone and saline are essentially radio-opaque. This means that X-rays do not pass through them, so they appear on the films as solid white areas. Some new implants being tested allow X-rays to pass through them and are, therefore, more useful with mammograms. Mammograms can confirm the presence of a gross rupture if globules of silicone gel are seen clearly outside the normal and expected round contour of the implant. They are useful in locating and assessing lumps or suspicious areas within breast tissue itself. This is more true as women age, since, with time, there is relatively more fat within the breast. This provides better contrast with breast tissue and calcified areas that may warrant further investigation. In implant assessment, however, mammograms tend to be only minimally useful.

This is also true of a sonogram (ultrasound) of the breast. This test is performed by placing a probe that looks like a small microphone on the breast. The probe bounces high-frequency sound waves off the breast and implant and then "reads" the contour mapped out by the pattern it generates. Ultrasound is particularly useful in locating masses and in distinguishing solid ones from fluid-filled ones. It typically provides information that suggests certain problems, such as the presence of silicone or fluid outside the normal confines of the implant. It is somewhat non-specific; i.e., it shows things that may not be clearly identified, and it may misread a fold as a leak. When combined with physical exam, however, both mammograms and sonograms add information. Because they are relatively simple and inexpensive to perform, these tests are used widely.

A more involved procedure is a CT Scan. This computerized X-ray image is obtained by having the patient lie down inside a machine which then passes repeatedly over the specific portions of the body to be assessed. Although the level of detail is significantly better than a mammogram, the CT Scan has many of the same limitations, as the X-rays still do not penetrate the implant itself. Despite the sophisticated nature of this test, specific locations on and around the implants can be missed due to technical considerations. If a small area of concern is between those passes (called "cuts"), it may not appear on the exam. It is, additionally, a more expensive test than either of the above. For these reasons, it is not typically part of implant assessment.

At present, the most accurate non-invasive examination of breast implants is the MRI, or Magnetic Resonance Imaging, when used with a breast coil. MRIs use a powerful magnet to help create their images, and patients with certain metal implants (including inner ear, pacemakers, and clips that may have been used in previous surgeries) should not undergo this test. The information provided by this test is by far the most useful of those described in this chapter. It is often possible to visualize both the outside and the inside of the implant(s), allowing a detailed examination of the implants.

The MRI takes about 15–20 minutes, and as with the CT Scan, the patient is essentially inside the machine. During this test the patient kneels forward onto her chest while placing her breasts directly into a specially formed adapter that is part of the machine. About 5% of patients are claustrophobic enough to be uncomfortable during the exam. Discussions ahead of time and, when needed, the use of anti-anxiety medications, help alleviate these concerns. "Open" forms of MRIs provide less clear images and are therefore less useful.

If a problem is identified, the question then becomes what to do about it. Needle biopsies are rarely used in this situation as the risk of damaging the implant is too high. Consequently, the safest and most definitive method of examining a lump or suspicious area is an open biopsy (see Chapter 22).

No test is 100% accurate. There have been cases where implants reported to be ruptured on the basis of non-invasive studies have been found, at surgery, to be completely intact. Once the surgery has begun, it is generally, though not always, necessary to remove them even if they weren't ruptured. The surgery itself can damage the implant mechanically, or the risk of postoperative infection may warrant their removal. A number of perfectly good silicone implants have been removed because of this scenario, essentially for no good reason.

In summary, women who are concerned about their implants do not, at present, have the simple, accurate, and inexpensive way of assessing them that would be desirable. In view of the worldwide popularity of breast implants, this is as surprising as it is unfortunate; it is hoped that more practical imaging techniques will become available.

CHAPTER 20

Breast Lifts and Reductions

Breast lifts and reductions are discussed together because they are similar procedures. The difference is the amount of breast tissue removed. When skin and a small amount of breast tissue (by one standard, less than 300 grams — about 30 ounces) are removed the procedure is termed a lift, or mastopexy. When more breast tissue than that is removed, it is termed a breast reduction.

In each situation, the relative excesses of skin and breast tissue need to be determined. If the overall breast size is more or less acceptable, and the only problem is too much sagging, then the appropriate procedure is a lift. In this procedure the breast and nipple position are raised, excess skin is removed and the entire skin "envelope" of the breast is tightened. In most cases, the size of the areola (the dark area around the nipple) is reduced. A breast lift improves the appearance of the breasts and diminishes the "ravages of time," not to mention pregnancy and/or weight loss. Neither this nor any other procedure inherently reverses the aging process and the effects of time or gravity, which seems to get back to work almost immediately. Still, whatever degree of sagging may remain or recur after a lift is much less than it would have been without the surgery.

The results of a breast reduction are even more dramatic. In addition to the benefits achieved with a lift, the reduction in size can have a major impact on the patient's quality of life. Symptoms associated with large breasts include neck, shoulder, and back pain, rashes, painful bra strap grooving, fatigue, and the inability to exercise or to sleep on one's back (breathing is difficult in this position due to the weight of the breasts). These patients often have problems getting clothes to fit. Many women have to buy two different sizes: one for the top, a second for the bottom. Simply losing weight, even when possible, does not adequately reduce the size of the breasts. This is due to the makeup of breasts: skin, fat, and breast (i.e., glandular) tissue itself. Reducing the fat may help somewhat, but is rarely enough to produce an improvement in the symptoms noted above. The glandular elements prevent an adequate reduction of breast size with weight loss, which is largely loss of fat. It is discouraging for these women to lose weight, only to see that their body proportions remain essentially unchanged or, worse, that other areas get smaller faster than their breasts. Conversely, after breast reduction surgery, patients are often more motivated to lose weight and to keep it off. Aside from any psychological explanation, patients see that weight loss can actually produce the body shape and proportions they want. Most women who undergo this procedure are extremely pleased with the surgery and the effect it has on their life.

A wide variety of breast reduction procedures has been described. For a number of reasons, surgeons often select the technique to be used based on the amount of reduction anticipated. All of the procedures leave scars in one or more areas of the breast. It is almost always necessary to have a scar around the areola (the dark area around the nipple). In most cases, there is also a vertical scar that extends from the lowest point of the areola (the six o'clock position) down to the crease that goes underneath the breast (called the "inframammary crease"). In many cases, there must also be a horizontal scar within a portion of this crease itself. The larger the breast, the more likely one will need the complete scar pattern, which is essentially shaped like an anchor. The presence of scars on the breasts (often from previous breast biopsies) may preclude the use of specific techniques.

The variant that produces the least amount of scarring is called a concentric mastopexy or reduction, which leaves a circular scar around the areola. It is most useful for small lifts and when an implant is being used in addition to the lift. The implant helps to fill out the breast, thereby reducing the amount of skin that would otherwise need to be removed in tightening the breast. Despite the minimal scars it leaves, this technique has drawbacks. For one, the degree of lift it can accomplish is limited, restricting its use primarily to small lifts. In addition, the breast shape it produces is flat centrally (including the areola), rather than conical. Finally, the circular scars can become thick and wide with time, and the areolas tend to spread out (due to tension); in larger reductions this scar may spread to an unacceptable degree. For these reasons, this technique is not used as often as one might think.

In reducing and repositioning breast tissue, a surgical configuration termed a "pedicle" is created. This refers to the manner in which the central portion of the breast, including the nipple, is shaped. Pedicles based on nearly all portions of the breast have been described, but most procedures in use today are based on either superior (upper) or inferior (lower) pedicles. In general, larger reductions can be accomplished more safely using the inferior pedicle technique, particularly with respect to how far the nipple is lifted. Furthermore, there is less disruption of the breast tissue, specifically the connection between the glands and the ducts of the nipple, with an inferior pedicle breast reduction than with a superior pedicle procedure. For this reason, many surgeons feel that there is better preservation of sensation as well as an increased likelihood of breast feeding postoperatively with the inferior pedicle procedure than with the superior pedicle procedures. Breast feeding is discussed in more detail below.

One popular technique is a relatively recent addition to the procedures currently available. Madeleine Lejour, a Belgian plastic surgeon, developed a technique in which the horizontal limb, i.e., the scar that lies horizontally within the crease underneath the breast, can be eliminated. This superior pedicle variant, often termed a "vertical mammaplasty," produces a breast lift or reduction in which the only scars are those around the areola and a vertical scar. The resultant shape, akin to a lollipop, is a significant improvement over the complete scar pattern that is required in most breast reductions.

Naturally, there are some trade-offs with this technique, particularly with large breasts. The horizontal scar is normally used to remove excess skin lying horizontally along the crease under the breast. Not having this means that this skin must be addressed in a way other than direct excision. This technique makes use of the skin's ability to contract. The excess skin is bunched together in a vertical direction. As the breast settles after the surgery and the skin contracts, the bunching becomes less pronounced. Breasts reduced in this manner may heal with somewhat widened scars. Occasionally, small surgical revisions are needed several months postoperatively to remove some excess skin and/or improve the appearance of the vertical scar. The benefit of this procedure (i.e., no horizontal scar, or minimal if a revision is required) is so desirable that the vertical mammaplasty is often an excellent choice.

In extremely large breasts the blood supply of the pedicle, which supplies the nipple, may be unreliable. In these cases, the nipples are placed into their new positions as grafts. Consequences of this technique include pigmentary (color) changes of the nipple and areola and some loss of sensation of the nipple, since areolas replaced in this fashion do not regain sensation as well as with pedicled reductions. Nevertheless these patients, because of the dramatic results and degree of relief they obtain, are almost universally delighted with their surgery.

Another concern with this surgery is the potential for breast feeding. There is relatively little conclusive scientific data concerning this issue. One study examined breast feeding after inferior pedicle breast reduction.[14] It found that

---

[14] Harris, L. Is breast feeding possible after reduction mammaplasty? *Plast. Reconstr. Surg.* 89:836, 1992.

100% of patients lactated after becoming pregnant and that all patients who wanted to breast feed were able to do so. This may not apply to all techniques, however. As noted above, the inferior pedicle leaves the nipple directly attached to and effectively centralized on much of the remaining breast tissue, which may explain its suitability for breast feeding. In other techniques, the connections between the breast glands and the nipple postoperatively are more circuitous. Another study concluded that the more breast tissue removed during the surgery, the less likely that patients would be able to breast feed afterwards. There may be different explanations for this, but since breast reduction disrupts the anatomy of the breast, it is not entirely surprising. While a patient may not be able to breast feed after a reduction, most patients can do so. (Some women, even without having had surgery, are not able to breast feed successfully.) Interestingly, the changes seen after pregnancy (primarily sagging and the need for a small reduction, if at all) lend themselves particularly well to correction with the superior pedicle technique. Breast feeding tends to be less of a concern in these patients. Younger and pre-pregnancy patients are more likely to benefit from the inferior pedicle procedure which, appropriately, may be better suited for future breast feeding. Nevertheless, this potential trade-off is among those that should be taken into account when considering a breast reduction.

CHAPTER 21

Complications of Breast Reductions

Patients are extremely satisfied with this procedure. Most cases heal with few or no significant side effects, although the complications noted previously can occur with this procedure, too. Changes in sensation are common, but, interestingly, the sensation is often better after the surgery than before. Prospective breast reduction patients typically have less than average nipple sensation. This is presumably because the excess weight of the breasts stretches and dulls the nerves. With the tissues under less stretch after the reduction, sensation is improved. The improved body image that is produced by the breast reduction may also contribute to the improved sensation, and to the increase in pleasure derived from the reduced and reshaped breasts.

Asymmetry (i.e., one side or part of the body looking different from the other) is common in general. Most people are not completely symmetrical naturally. This applies to all parts of the body, but is often most noticeable on the face and on the breasts. While every attempt is made to preserve and to produce symmetry with a breast reduction, it is not always possible to do so. Preoperative differences in, for example, the size or width of the breasts and/or the relative positions of the nipples contribute to this problem. Slight differences are common after this surgery and do not normally require intervention postoperatively. More significant asymmetry can usually be improved with a minor surgical procedure, often done in the doctor's office.

Some degree of scarring is an unavoidable consequence of this procedure. In most cases, the location and quality of the scars are well within an acceptable range, particularly in view of the benefits achieved. Even in cases where the scarring turns out to be less than ideal the improvement in their quality of life is so dramatic that patients are usually satisfied with the overall results. Treatment of unsightly and/or painful scars generally consists of topical therapy (massage, pressure, stretching, etc.), injections of anti-inflammatory medications (such as steroids — not the type that increase muscle bulk!), and scar revisions. These are procedures, designed to improve the appearance of scars, in which the undesirable scars are removed and the skin is resewn with several layers of sutures under minimal or no tension. Steroids are often injected during and after this procedure to help prevent the scars from reforming.

There may also be a change in color of the areolas. This occurs most commonly with the graft procedure used on the largest breasts. Areolas may be lighter or darker than they were preoperatively. In most cases the color eventually returns to normal; in some cases it does not. Medical grade tattooing, similar to what is used for breast reconstruction, is an option for these patients.

Finally, a rare complication is delayed healing with widened scars. This is when portions of the skin heal by gradual replacement with scar tissue and contraction of the surrounding skin, rather than healing normally. This usually affects the skin underneath the breast, but it can include the nipple and areola, in which case reconstruction and/or tattooing may be necessary. Excessive bleeding, infection and conditions that reduce blood flow, such as diabetes, circulatory disorders, and tobacco use, predispose to this complication.

CHAPTER 22

Breast Lumps, Cancer, and Reconstruction after Mastectomy

Breast lumps are common, and fortunately, most are benign (i.e., not cancerous). Nevertheless, finding one is a nerve-wracking experience. Lumps can be solid, filled with fluid (called a cyst), or a combination. They can persist, or they can appear and then disappear. Those that persist can stay the same or can change in size and/or consistency, often related to the menstrual or hormonal status. They may be familial; it is common for women with breast lumps to report that female relatives have them also.

Breast lumps can occur among patients who have had previous breast surgery of any kind, including breast enlargements, lifts, reductions, and excision of breast masses. These lumps are often deep to or near scars on the skin. They can form as part of the healing process or around bits of suture material, and normally they consist of scar tissue. Although even more likely to be benign than in a patient who has not had any breast surgery, even these lumps must be investigated. Plastic surgeons often take care of these patients and perform the biopsies if indicated, particularly if a breast implant is involved, to avoid risking damage to the implant.

Breast lumps should not be ignored, as the possibility of cancer needs to be excluded. The initial surveillance and management of breast lumps is often undertaken by a woman's obstetrician or gynecologist and consists of medical history, physical examination, and non-invasive tests. If the mass does not disappear and is suspicious, it needs to be assessed more directly. If the lump is a cyst, an examination of the fluid may provide a diagnosis. This procedure, called "aspiration," is done by inserting a needle through the skin (under local anesthesia) and into the mass to withdraw a sample of the fluid, which is then examined by a laboratory. If the mass is solid, if it does not disappear after aspiration (as should happen with a cyst), or if examination of the cystic fluid is non-diagnostic (i.e., unclear), a biopsy is usually recommended. A biopsy is the surgical removal of a lump for examination by a pathologist to exclude cancer. It should be performed if there are suspicious findings on non-invasive tests like mammograms (X-rays of the breast) and ultrasound (which can distinguish between solid and fluid-filled masses), if breast lumps do not disappear (usually within two months of having been identified), or if there are particularly worrisome lumps. An exception may be if the woman has a history of multiple lumps, all of which have been benign on biopsy, and chooses to observe the progress of the mass with regular screening and physical exams. Biopsies can be performed by inserting a special needle (a "needle" biopsy) or through a direct surgical procedure (an "open" biopsy).

If cancer is diagnosed, it is removed or destroyed, usually by surgery. Further treatment is typically carried out by a breast or general surgeon, often a cancer specialist. There are several different procedures that can be used to remove breast cancer. These include a lumpectomy (removal of the lump with only a small amount of surrounding breast tissue), a quadrantectomy (removal of the lump with about the quarter of breast tissue in which it is situated), and a mastectomy (removal of the entire breast). The nipple, as well as some axillary lymph nodes, may need to be removed, depending on the size and location of the mass. Since breast cancer has a tendency to be present in several parts of the breast at one time or in both breasts, additional therapies are often indicated. These include radiotherapy (X-ray or radiation therapy) and chemotherapy (drugs given to reduce or eliminate the tumor), each of which is administered under the direction of one or more specialists. A large amount of literature on these subjects is available in libraries, bookstores, and from other sources.[15]

If desired, the breast can be reconstructed after a mastectomy. Breast reconstruction has two goals: to recreate (1) the breast mound and (2) the nipple and areola. Because of the skin shortage that results from a mastectomy, it is often nearly impossible to recreate the mound without adding or stretching some tissue, although some techniques of removing the tumor spare more skin and tissue than others. While the volume of a breast mound (i.e., the way it fills a bra cup) may be recreated adequately by inserting an implant under the muscle, the shape that it produces, particularly out of a bra, often does not match the conical shape and slight droop of a normal breast. This is even more of a problem for young patients and whenever the skin is relatively tight. Depending on the size and shape of the remaining breast, it may be advantageous to stretch the skin and muscle on the side being reconstructed by inserting a tissue expander. This is a hollow silicone bag, similar to what is used for a saline implant, that is inserted empty or partially filled. It is then expanded periodically over the next several weeks or months by injecting saline (a minor office procedure requiring only local anesthesia). Once the skin and tissues are stretched sufficiently, the expander is replaced with a permanent implant. Sometimes the opposite breast is modified to maintain symmetry. This may be a lift, a reduction, the insertion of an implant, or a combination of a lift with an implant.

Another approach is to add tissue taken from a different part of the body. Most of these procedures eliminate the need for an implant, including any problems in the future related to the implant; with some, an implant is still required. The most popular of these is called the "TRAM Flap" (Transverse Rectus Abdominus Muscle). In this procedure, skin and fat

---

[15] An excellent and encyclopedic text is *Dr. Susan Love's Breast Book*, Second Edition, Reading, MA, The Addison Wesley Publishing Company, 1995.

from the lower stomach, based on the blood supply within the rectus abdominus muscle (the "abs"), are moved up to the breast and fashioned into a breast shape. Ideally suited for women who have excess skin and fat on the lower abdomen, the TRAM can produce outstanding results. An added benefit is that, in removing the abdominal tissue, a tummy tuck is performed. Other procedures use tissue from the back or buttocks region (which requires microsurgery to reattach the blood supply to the tissue). Not all patients are equally good candidates for all procedures. Diabetes, tobacco smoking, obesity, and other medical conditions may preclude their safe use. In addition, the scarring, recovery, and risks are more extensive than with an implant alone. Nevertheless, it is possible to recreate the breast mound, eliminating the need to wear prostheses (artificial breasts that are held within custom-made bras, bathing suits, etc.).

The second stage is the reconstruction of the nipple and areola. This is done through a combination of small skin procedures, skin grafting, and/or medical-grade tattooing. In general, the results achieved with these procedures do not last as long as people would like, requiring subsequent procedures such as repeat tattooing. Because of this, as well as the realization that it may not be possible to recreate the entire breast adequately, some patients are content with the reconstruction of the breast mound alone.

Breast reconstruction can be performed at the time of the mastectomy or at a later date. There are advantages to its being performed at the initial surgery, although it does increase the length of the surgery. Having the plastic surgeon observe the precise amount and pattern of breast tissue that is removed increases the likelihood that the reconstructed breast will more closely match the breast it is designed to replace, particularly when tissue from the patient's own body is being used. In addition, completing the reconstruction before the normal scarring and contraction of healing has set in helps the tissues remain soft. Sometimes a tissue expander is inserted at the initial procedure and expanded later. Equally good results, however, can be achieved with delayed reconstructions.

Prevention, early detection, and research for a cure remain the critical aspects in the fight against breast cancer. Improved techniques of ablation (cancer removal) and breast reconstruction have lessened — if only a little — the trauma these patients go through. It is hoped that progress in the fight against breast cancer will ultimately render breast reconstruction obsolete.

Section 3

Liposuction

CHAPTER 23

What is Liposuction and Why Does It Work?

Liposuction is the permanent removal of fat using a suction technique. It is a contouring procedure that is used to reshape specific areas of the body. Many people are unhappy about the fat they have on one or more parts of their body, and liposuction is now the most commonly performed cosmetic surgery in the United States. Plastic surgery that reshapes the body by removing or altering fat is termed "lipoplasty."

Nearly every part of the body has been successfully treated with liposuction. For women, the most common areas treated are the thighs ("saddle-bags"), hips, stomach, and neck (often instead of a facelift, particularly in younger patients); for men, the "love handles" on the waist, the stomach, chest (including male breasts or "gynecomastia"), and neck. Liposuction is frequently combined with other operations, such as facelifts, breast reductions, tummy tucks, and a variety of reconstructive procedures, to maximize their effect.

Using one or more small, hidden incisions, a cannula, or hollow tube, is inserted under the skin. The cannula typically measures about 1/8 to 3/8 inch in diameter, and is open at both ends. One end is connected to a suction machine, which provides the vacuum necessary to perform the procedure. The tip of the other end, which comes in a variety of configurations and shapes, is inserted under the skin and then placed within the collections of fat. Once the vacuum is applied, fat is removed, a little at a time, wherever the tip of the cannula is placed. The body is literally sculpted; more fat is taken from the areas that require it most, and less from the surrounding areas. During the procedure, the surgeon uses one hand to hold the cannula and the other to feel the skin and to decide how much fat needs to be removed from each area. The patient is normally marked prior to surgery; a pen is used to circle the areas that will be treated, including the most prominent spots. The planned procedure is discussed in advance, but the final determinations and decisions are made at the time of surgery. At the completion of the surgery, sutures may be placed to close the incisions. Usually, although not always, these are absorbable (dissolving) sutures that will not need to be removed. With some techniques and/or sites on the body, the incisions are not sutured but are left open to allow drainage; these incisions heal spontaneously over the next several weeks or months. This is discussed in further detail below.

One of the major advantages of this procedure is that there are essentially no visible scars. This is because the incisions are tiny to begin with (most measure about 1/8 to 1/2 inch in length), and they are placed whenever possible in natural skin creases or folds, such as under the buttocks or within the umbilicus (belly button). Under most circumstances, they are nearly invisible. For example, liposuction of the hips, outer thighs, and inner thighs can often be performed through a *single* 1/2 inch incision (on each side) that is completely hidden within the fold underneath the buttocks (infragluteal). All scars are permanent, and the specific characteristics of a scar are somewhat unpredictable, but the virtual absence of noticeable scars is one of the most beneficial aspects of liposuction. Scars from previous operations do not necessarily preclude a liposuction; in fact, they can be used as insertion sites for the liposuction cannulas. The specific sites and placement of the incisions are discussed later, in the chapters that detail each region individually.

Because of the anatomy of the regions involved, it is normally the deep fat that is removed, while leaving a layer of superficial fat under the skin. It has been shown that there are structural differences between the superficial and the deep fat layers, and they behave differently, both at the time of surgery and during the healing process. The superficial fat layer is dense and firm, and is somewhat more difficult to remove with liposuction. By contrast, the deep layer is looser and much more amenable to liposuction. Different anatomical regions have different proportions of superficial and deep fat, and the surgery must be tailored individually taking this into account.

The final result of liposuction depends both on the amount of fat removed and on the ability of the skin to redrape into its new contour (see Chapter 27 for a discussion of the skin). After the surgery, there is swelling and bruising to varying degrees that subside as part of the healing. The absorption of swelling and the redraping of the skin can take several weeks or months. Improvement in some areas is often visible immediately after surgery and much of the effect is noted by about 6 weeks, but the final appearance may not be "set" for up to 6 months after surgery. I tell my patients that they can expect to have 80% of the result in 4–6 weeks, 95% by three months, and that the last bit may take the full six months. Interestingly, this gradual transformation following a liposuction can help to keep the procedure relatively private. Postoperatively, the body shrinks over a period of weeks to months (hidden under your regular clothes) suggesting a remarkable weight loss through, presumably, diet and exercise alone. The final result can then be revealed whenever —and however—you want.

Although the final results of liposuction are not evident for several months, the effects are dramatic and can be apparent much sooner. Many women have been able to go from, for example, a size 10 to a 6. One woman wore a size 26 jeans preoperatively; three weeks after her surgery, size 14 was loose and she had lost 5 inches from her hip circumference. Another patient lost 8 inches in 8 weeks. A 53-year-old woman lost five inches from the circumference of each thigh. Liposuction enabled a 44-year-old woman to stay under water when trying to dive while snorkeling without wearing a weight belt, which she had previously needed (Patient # 50). Finally, several weeks after his liposuction, a 26-year-old man put on a pair of pants that had been snug and closed his belt at the usual hole. As he reached for his jacket, his pants slipped down to his ankles.

Although extended by advances in surgical techniques, there is a limit to the amount of fat that can be removed safely at a single procedure, and liposuction is not a treatment for obesity. Dramatic changes in the relative proportions of one's body can be accomplished by removing less than a pound of fat. Fat is one of the lightest tissues in the body (it is lighter than bone, muscle, or skin), so a pound is a relatively large volume. Liposuction is a contouring procedure and most people achieve excellent results with a single procedure. For large amounts, however, more than one procedure may be required.

Liposuction is performed in anatomical locations that do not have major blood vessels or nerves, and the majority of what is removed is fat. Some blood is, nevertheless, removed at the same time. This helps explain the restrictions on the amount of "fat" that can be removed at any one time. Certain techniques reduce the amount of blood that is lost during the procedure (see below).

Liposuction is not a treatment for cellulite. Although nearly everyone knows what you mean when you say "cellulite" (the "cottage cheese" appearance of the surface of the outer thigh, for example), it is not much different biologically from regular fat.[16] This fat, however, is located right under the skin, which is why it is so noticeable. Since liposuction is most effective on the deep fat, cellulite normally is not adequately treated by liposuction alone. It may become less noticeable after liposuction, however, due to the contraction of the skin and fat, as well as the fact that the entire area protrudes less. Reducing the "bulk" of the thighs can improve the appearance of the legs, even with the

---

[16] One report concluded that the appearance of cellulite was actually due to a weakness in the supporting connective tissue, rather than of the fat itself. Ship, A. Cellulite: morphology and biochemistry. Presented at ASAPS Meeting, New York, May 1997.

persistence of some cellulite. A slim leg, with or without cellulite, is generally considered to be more attractive than a heavier leg. Cellulite remains an unsolved problem. If the thighs are nearly ideal and cellulite is the only thing being treated on the leg (i.e., there is no contour deformity), liposuction is not an adequate treatment.

Some areas of fat are not accessible to liposuction. For example, the shape of one's stomach may be due largely to fat that is deep to the muscles. This is particularly common for men and can also occur with neck fat, i.e., fat under the chin. Normally this can be determined before surgery by doing a "pinch" test. Briefly, while tensing the muscles, the skin and fat of various regions of the body are pinched gently. In areas where a lot of fat is identified directly under the skin (i.e., between the skin and the muscles), improvement can be expected with a liposuction. If relatively little fat is identified in this layer, the region may not be amenable to correction with liposuction. Additionally, if there is a large amount of excess skin, procedures that tighten the skin, with or without liposuction, may be required.

Finally, liposuction can also be used to remove localized collections of benign fatty growths, called "lipomas," that occur under a variety of conditions. Most often they appear singly and are located on the arms or back. In some cases lipomas may be a consequence of a medical condition, such as Cushing's syndrome. Liposuction allows the removal of large growths through small incisions, thereby avoiding large scars.

CHAPTER 24

Why Won't Diet and Exercise Work Just as Well?

Diet and exercise are extremely important in general, not only in terms of overall health, but also with respect to fat. Eating appropriately is considered the most important factor, but the total amount of fat in one's body is decreased most effectively by controlling the intake of calories (food) and, at the same time, exercising regularly. Even when successful, however, the specific areas of fat reduction are not optional, i.e., you do not get to pick the locations from which the fat will be removed. When weight is lost via diet and exercise, it is lost in proportion to the total amount of fat in the body. Most of the loss is from the areas that have most of the fat.

These areas, however, may not be the ones of greatest concern to the patient; proportionate fat loss is not always desirable. Fat is often lost from, for example, a woman's face and breasts (leading to a loss of total breast volume, i.e., cup size) long before "enough" is lost from the thighs or stomach. Only a superhuman, unsustainable effort could result in an adequate loss of fat from these areas, and the effects on the appearance of the face (i.e., thinner, with more lines!) and the rest of the body would not necessarily be desirable. Liposuction is almost a kind of "target" or "spot" dieting; you get to pick where you want the reductions made. It enables you to reverse the cycle of losing it just where you'd like to keep it, and vice versa. It may be possible to retain the desired shape of the face and chest (for example) while still reducing the thighs and hips. If the desired shape can be achieved and maintained through diet and/or exercise alone, then having surgery makes little sense.

It is common for people to try to reduce one specific area (e.g., stomach or thighs) by concentrating their exercising on that spot. Ironically, such "focused" exercising of an area can actually increase its size. As the muscles gain tone and become firm, their bulk also increases. This makes the entire area larger. For example, doing situps may help you lose weight (from all over your body) and improve stomach tone and strength, but it is likely that the waist measurement will actually increase. If the goal is a flat tummy, the ideal regimen is a combination of controlled caloric intake, general aerobic exercise, avoidance of intensive situps and other stomach exercises, and if indicated, liposuction of the stomach. The many patients who have spent time and money exercising their stomachs and seeing minimal improvement, only to achieve immediate and permanent results with liposuction, can attest to that. One woman, a 35-year-old health club executive, had been trying to get rid of the "pouch" on her stomach for 3 years. This included daily workouts on her own, twice-weekly sessions with a personal trainer, and yearly visits to a spa — all with minimal results. If anything, she said, her stomach seemed bigger since she started doing all those situps. Frustrated, she took a friend's suggestion and underwent a liposuction of her stomach — along with her hips and thighs. Within a few weeks she was showing off her trim new shape. Her trainer was at a loss to explain her pupil's sudden improvement, and her friends at the spa were amazed at how much better she looked that year.

Furthermore, the playing field is not level. The amount of body fat as a percentage of one's total weight actually increases with time. For example, a 21-year-old man has an average of 13% of his weight as fat, but that increases to 26% by age 50. For a woman, that number increases from 25% at age 21 to 29% at age 50.[17] Not only does the percentage of fat change with time, but so does the distribution of fat on the body. This is the

[17] Chumlea WC. Adipocytes and adiposity in adults. *Amer. Jour. Clin. Nutr.* 34:1798, 1981.

beginning of the dreaded "middle age spread," when the weight that one carries shifts noticeably toward the middle of the body. The changes begin before middle age; often in the late 30s or early 40s. With increased fat deposition on the hips and stomach, a thin-waisted figure becomes one with a more squared or boxy shape. Hormonal changes contribute to this phenomenon. In most clothing, particularly the more fashionable and previously flattering, this shape is difficult to camouflage. The "matronly" look is largely characterized by this appearance of the waist and hips; liposuction of these areas makes the look more youthful. When shopping for outfits after a liposuction, patients may no longer need to go to one rack for the top, and another for the bottom.

Interestingly, one's body image can be harder to alter than the body itself. It is not unusual to hear that patients, upon entering a clothing store, still head directly for the racks of their presurgical size. This may last for a year or more; long after the body itself has adjusted to its new size. This ambiguity does not manifest itself on the body. The effects of liposuction are quantifiable, precise, dramatic, and permanent. No regimen of diet and/or exercise can match the effectiveness and the specificity — losing fat permanently where, and only where, one wants — of liposuction.

CHAPTER 25

Why Doesn't the Fat Come Back?

The distribution of fat in the body is often set early in life. Many factors contribute to the shape of one's body; among the most important are heredity, food consumption (both as a child and as an adult), metabolic rate, and one's level of activity. The total number of fat cells in the body remains relatively stable (unless, according to one study, there is a weight gain of at least 170% of the ideal body weight).[18] Once a fat cell has been formed, it is very difficult to remove it under normal circumstances.

As leftover calories accumulate and are converted to fat, existing fat cells grow larger and weight is gained. If adequate steps are taken to reverse this process (limiting caloric intake, increasing the level of activity so as to burn up more fat, etc.), the fat cells diminish in size. The fat cells may empty almost completely, but generally they do not disappear. (Studies have shown that fat cells actually can disappear under conditions of starvation or prolonged fasting, but that is not relevant to this discussion.) The fat cells remain as empty sacs; unfortunately, they can be refilled easily at any time. This helps to explain why it is so difficult to keep weight off once the initial loss has been achieved with traditional weight-loss programs: The cells continue to exist and reaccumulate the fat as soon as the person reverts to eating more and/or exercising less. There are other factors (habits, activity, psychology, etc.) that contribute to the immensely complicated question of why people find it so difficult to lose weight and, perhaps even more so, to maintain the loss. Nevertheless, this

[18] Markman, B. Anatomy and physiology of adipose tissue. *Clinics in Plastic Surgery.* Vol. 16, Philadelphia, PA, W.B. Saunders, 1989.

anatomic feature of fat cells is a contributing factor.

Liposuction is the permanent removal of fat. The fat that is removed is actually a mass of fat cells. Once removed, these fat cells can't grow back — they're gone. This produces a permanent change in the relative distribution of fat in the body. While small in proportion to the total amount of fat in the body, the fat removed during a liposuction can make a striking change in the relative relationships of the visible, external fat of the body. Having liposuction does not prevent future weight gain. If one overeats (or lowers the level of activity, or both) after this procedure, one can gain weight. Excess fat, once created from the leftover calories consumed, is deposited into the many remaining fat cells throughout the body. Liposuction does not alter this process.

After a liposuction, however, there are two major differences. First, if fat is added, it will arrange itself in a different distribution throughout the body than it would have before the liposuction. For example, if, before surgery, a woman who gained a few pounds noted that most of it would go to her thighs and hips, then after surgery (i.e., liposuction of the thighs and hips), the fat will typically go to different areas, such as the stomach, chest, or arms. One patient who underwent liposuction of her thighs and knees (but not her stomach or hips) told me that whenever she gained five pounds before her procedure, a certain pair of jeans became tight at the thighs; when she gains weight now, they became tight at the waist.

This pattern of subsequent contour alteration indicates both that the liposuction permanently changes the relative distribution of fat in the body, and that one has no choice as to where the additional fat will be distributed. This can be advantageous; about 20% of women who put on a little weight following a liposuction of the stomach, hips, and thighs report that their breasts got larger! In view of the above explanation, this phenomenon is understandable.

The natural conclusion is to do liposuction of the stomach, hips, and thighs together routinely, and I usually recommend exactly that. The stomach, hips, and thighs are often considered a single anatomic unit, even if one of the components is more troublesome than the others. Recontouring all the areas within a unit maintains this balance and helps prevent future disproportionate weight gain. Liposuction, therefore, is typically done on not only the target area(s), but on other, related areas.

Despite all the time spent trying to reduce one's weight through diet and exercise, the real issue is often the contour. The patient may (or may not) step on a scale every day, but what other people see is the relative shape, not the absolute weight. This was demonstrated by a patient who underwent a mini-tummy tuck and liposuction of her stomach, hips, and thighs. Several months later she showed off her striking new shape. As we finished talking, she casually mentioned that she had put on eight pounds since her surgery. Puzzled, I asked her why that was. "Because I've been eating like a pig," she replied, adding that despite her weight gain, everybody was telling her how fabulous she looked. This underscores the importance of the relative contour rather than the absolute weight. While most people work hard to look their best by keeping their weight at or below what it was preoperatively, and are successful at it, the overall appearance of the body remains enhanced even if a few extra pounds are added after the surgery.

Another difference after surgery is psychological. This aspect is not limited to liposuction, but is seen with other procedures such as breast reductions and tummy tucks. For many people, the surgery itself provides the stimulus needed to achieve and maintain the weight loss; it supplies the extra psychological boost, or incentive, that was missing previously. Having taken the trouble to undergo the surgery, patients often feel that they want to do everything possible to maximize the results. One patient had three pounds of fat removed during a liposuction, and then went on to lose another six through diet and aggressive exercise. Her dress size dropped from a 6–7 (top) and 8–9 (bottom) to a 4 after the liposuction and subsequent weight loss. She later commented, "I would never have been able to do that if I hadn't had the liposuction." In the fight against fat, willpower is a potent ally.

CHAPTER 26

Surgical Technique: Cannulas, Fluid, and Incisions

Many factors go into producing a good result from liposuction. Appropriate patient selection, surgical expertise, and a variety of technical considerations, including the number and location of incisions, size of cannulas, use of vasoconstricting fluid, etc., are all important. No single technique, instrument, or piece of equipment necessarily guarantees success and a good cosmetic result; instead, it is the combination of the above that produces the best result.

Surgical techniques vary widely, and so do the things that are done in conjunction with, and that modify, the surgery itself. Over the twenty or so years that liposuction has been in wide usage, many different approaches, whether directly surgical or in preparation for the surgery, have been employed. There have been several general trends. One concerns the size (the diameter) of the cannula that is used to perform the liposuction. This may refer to either the internal or the external diameters of a cannula. For example, a cannula with an external diameter of 6 millimeters (mm) typically has an internal diameter of about 4.5 mm (there are about 25 mm to an inch). Originally the cannulas were relatively large; i.e., an external diameter of about 8 to 10 mm, or just under half an inch. Using smaller cannulas has advantages: They are less likely to cause rippling and waves (i.e., visible evidence of the tracks the cannula has made), and they cause less trauma and therefore less postoperative discomfort. Over time the diameters of the cannulas used have become smaller, even though these cannulas reduce the amount of fat removed with each stroke. Most surgeons now use cannulas with external diameters that range from about 2 to 6 mm. The larger cannulas are often used for the deeper layers, and the smaller ones for the more superficial layers.

Originally, the procedure was done without preinjecting any fluids (now referred to as the "dry" technique). An incision was made in the skin, the cannula was inserted and fat was removed. Although effective, too much blood was lost with the fat, so steps were taken to reduce the blood loss. First, surgeons started preinjecting (i.e., several minutes before starting the surgery) some fluid that contained both local anesthesia and epinephrine (also called adrenaline), a chemical that, among other things, constricts blood vessels and decreases the amount of bleeding that is associated with the surgery. The addition of an anesthetic (usually lidocaine) provides some numbness and decreases the amount and level of sedation required during the procedure. This is now referred to as the "wet" technique and it decreases the blood loss associated with liposuction. Ironically, the dry technique is wet (i.e., bloody), while the wet technique is dry.

Over time, the type and amount of solution injected has evolved. Surgeons started injecting even more fluid, thereby decreasing the blood loss further; this is now referred to as "superwet." Another advantage of using increased amounts of fluid is that less anesthesia (i.e., sedation, whether intravenous or oral) is required than if less fluid is used. Yet another is that the fluid "softens" the tissues, which makes it easier and less traumatic for the cannulas to pass through them. Although the specific amount of solution that has to be injected in order to be called "wet" or "superwet" has been specified, the terms are used loosely. Each surgeon has his or her preferred amount and composition of this fluid, and it has never been completely standardized. It is common for surgeons to adjust the amount of fluid used depending on the case in question.

More recently, the term "tumescent" liposuction was

introduced. When a large amount of fluid is injected into the tissues prior to performing the liposuction, it may be termed tumescent, which means "swollen." According to the literal interpretation of the tumescent technique, the tissues are filled with enough fluid to be swollen and firm. Many factors influence the amount of fluid that is required to tumesce the tissues, including the size of the areas to be treated and the thickness and elasticity of the tissues. Exactly how much fluid has to be used in order to qualify as tumescent is debatable. One "formula" states that one injects whatever it takes to tumesce the tissues. Another is that an amount of fluid equal to the amount of fat one anticipates removing during the liposuction should be injected beforehand; others say twice or two and a half times that amount. The amount of fat actually removed, however, is not always the same as the amount that one anticipated. The strict use of this technique can mean quite a bit of fluid is injected; in some cases up to twenty liters (a liter is about a quart, so this amount represents about five gallons of fluid). Often a combination of subcutaneous and intravenous fluid is used to provide replacement. The tumescent technique does not per se imply the use of any specific sedation or general anesthesia. This technique can be used with local anesthesia alone, intravenous sedation, or regional or general anesthesia.

The fluid is injected subcutaneously, and although much of it is removed surgically during the procedure, not all of it is. Whatever is not removed in this manner must be absorbed by the body and then excreted. The absorption and subsequent excretion of large amounts of fluid can be stressful for the body, particularly the heart, lungs, and kidneys. Concern has been expressed that absorption of significant amounts of fluid could be dangerous. Additionally, there may be toxic phar- macologic effects from the absorption of epinephrine and lidocaine, particularly when large volumes have been injected. Blood levels may not even peak until twelve hours after injection. There are at least several reports that justify these concerns.[19] For this reason, many surgeons modify the amount of fluid they routinely inject, decreasing it to remain within a range that they feel is safe.

Another potential disadvantage of this technique is that the large amount of fluid injected may obscure the contour of the specific region being treated, making accurate assessment during the surgery that much more difficult. I generally agree with this, particularly with the removal of smaller amounts of fat and with thinner patients. Some surgeons, however, feel that tumescence makes contour abnormalities easier to treat. In any event, one surgeon's "tumescent" technique is another's "superwet." The use of fluid in liposuction is the subject of ongoing discussion in the literature.[20]

The combination of lidocaine and epinephrine, providing local pain relief and decreased bleeding, has been effective in changing the way this procedure is performed. In some cases, particularly when enough of this fluid is injected, procedures can be done without any intravenous sedation. Some surgeons, in fact, do all or most of their liposuction procedures using little or no sedation of any kind. Liposuction done in this manner normally requires the use of cannulas that are both thin and short, since thicker and/or longer cannulas would be too uncomfortable if used with local anesthesia alone. An advantage of longer cannulas is that they can be inserted from relatively fewer, more distant incisions and then maneuvered into positions appropriate for the surgery. This minimizes the number of incisions required to perform the surgery. Using shorter cannulas therefore requires more incisions — as discussed below, there are potential disadvantages to this.

Many surgeons feel that most anatomic regions can not be adequately contoured using local anesthesia alone, particu-

---

[19] *Allure,* September 1996, p 247, *The Bergen Record.* August 25, 1997, p A6, and Gilliland, MD. Tumescent liposuction complicated by pulmonary edema. *Plast. Reconstr. Surg.* 99:215, 1997.

[20] Rohrich RJ . The role of subcutaneous infiltration in suction-assisted lipoplasty: a review. *Plast. Reconstr. Surg.* 99: 514, 1997 and discussions of above. Similarly, Fodor, P. Wetting solutions in aspirative lipoplasty: a plea for safety in liposuction. *Aesth. Plast. Surg.* 19: 379, 1995, and Grazer, F. Complications of the tumescent formula for liposuction. *Plast. Reconstr. Surg.* 100:1893, 1997.

larly if multiple regions are being reduced during a single procedure, which is usually the case. This depends on the size of the region(s) being contoured and the amount of fat to be removed. This is that much more of an issue when multiple procedures (i.e., liposuction and eyelid surgery or breast enlargement) are being performed at the same time. This, too, is common. Furthermore, I have found that most patients do not even want to be fully awake and aware of what is going on during their procedure. They are very happy to go into a room, lie down on a table, enter a twilight zone, and wake up when it is over. For these reasons, most of my procedures are done using at least some degree of intravenous sedation. Smaller areas or less complete reductions of specific regions, however, can be satisfactorily treated and improved using local anesthesia alone.

Another issue is the placement (location) of the incisions, and whether they are sutured or left open. The incisions themselves are small (usually ranging from about 1/8 to 1/2 inch). Where they are placed depends partly on the manner in which they are used. I try to keep all or most of the incisions completely hidden, whenever possible, within existing skin creases, folds, the umbilicus (belly button) and pre-existing scars. There is no way to know exactly what any specific scar or insertion site will look like. The risk of leaving a visible and unaesthetic scar is significant enough so that, in my opinion, everything possible should be done to keep the incisions, and therefore the scars they produce, hidden. It has been said that scars are unnatural and unpredictable, and therefore undesirable.[21] Even if the incision heals well at the skin level, it can remain noticeable as the center of a sunken, depressed, and/or discolored area, creating an uneven contour that may be discernible through sheer clothes and bathing suits. This may be due to the trauma of the back and forth motion of the cannula as it passes repeatedly through the incision in the skin, to a slight over-resection (removal) of fat in that region since more cannula strokes occur there, or both. At least one

[21] D. Ralph Millard, MD.

incision (and therefore scar) is required in the vicinity of each area that is to be treated, although several areas can often be treated through one well-placed incision. For example, I typically use a *single* infragluteal incision (on each side) to perform liposuction on the hip, outer thigh, and inner thigh. Occasionally, depending on the size and locations of the areas to be recontoured, it is not possible to perform an adequate liposuction using such limited and distant incisions; in that case, others are required. Whenever possible, incisions are kept small and hidden in natural creases.

The next issue is whether or not the incisions should be closed (sutured). It might seem obvious that they should, but there are times when it makes sense not to do so. Some surgeons, in fact, routinely leave most or all of the incisions open. This has the advantage, depending on the exact placement of the incisions, of allowing drainage of fluid from the subcutaneous tissues (fluid refers both to some blood that inevitably is left behind by this procedure, as well as any of the fluid that was pre-injected). Increased evacuation and drainage of this fluid often leads to a more rapid and easier recovery. Fluid that remains within the body will be absorbed, but this process takes longer and is more uncomfortable than if the drainage is facilitated by leaving the incisions open.

There is, however, a good reason to close all but the smallest incisions with sutures (stitches), despite everything cited above. Depending on its location and size, an incision that has been sutured will normally produce a better (less noticeable) scar than one that has been left open. Since one is normally more concerned with the long-term and permanent results than with the first few days after the procedure, this approach usually makes more sense to me. Additionally, if the incisions are to be used for drainage, their placement must be adequate to allow that, i.e., they must be close enough and near the lower or central portion of the area to be treated to let gravity facilitate the drainage. If the incisions are hidden in inconspicuous locations, often at some distance from the surgical site (for the reasons noted above), they may be less effective in providing drainage. Finally, the drainage process itself is quite messy. For several days after the procedure, pinkish fluid comes out of the incisions; a lot at first, then gradually less over the next few days. A series of absorbent pads must be worn and changed frequently. They are often contained within a large, elastic, overalls-type garment.

Since the final appearance of the scars is an important consideration, I often recommend that many of the incisions, depending on their size and location, be closed with sutures. Some incisions can be left open without leaving noticeable scars. In the case of incisions placed within the umbilicus, within hair-bearing areas, or within existing scars, the resultant scars are so well hidden that their appearance becomes less of an issue and it is reasonable to take advantage of the benefits of leaving them open.

Another issue in liposuction is time, which is a factor in at least two aspects of the procedure. First, is the amount of time the surgeon waits between injecting the fluid and starting the procedure. It takes up to 20–30 minutes for the epinephrine to reach its full effect. Starting the surgery too soon after the subcutaneous injection reduces the vasoconstrictive effect of the fluid. The second aspect is how long it takes to do the procedure itself. The initial strokes of the cannula typically produce the purest fat. With time, the aspirate (the material removed) becomes increasingly blood-tinged. This is because there is less fat remaining in the region being treated and some of the epinephrine or tumescent effect wears off. Longer procedures can be associated with more blood loss. Also, the longer the procedure, the more anesthesia or sedation is required. Since side effects can be dose-related, it is preferable to use the least amount of anesthesia reasonable. In any event, there are advantages to performing the surgery in an expedient manner.

One of the attractions of liposuction is the way it can be individually tailored for each patient. This is much more so for liposuction than for any of the other procedures discussed in this book. Some patients prefer multiple small procedures done under local anesthesia, with or without light sedation and performed with multiple incisions; others prefer fewer procedures, fewer incisions, a single recovery period, and being less aware of the procedure itself. The nature of liposuction allows this "customizing," effectively matching specific modifications and variations of the procedure with patients' preferences.

CHAPTER 27

What Does the Skin Look Like After Liposuction?

The final result of a liposuction depends not only on the amount and distribution of the fat removed, but on the ability of the skin and remaining subcutaneous fat to redrape into a new contour. This phenomenon occurs naturally: With any form of significant weight loss after a significant gain, including pregnancy, the skin adapts to a new underlying framework and redrapes itself. This is essentially what happens with a liposuction. Fat is removed, leaving the skin and a supporting framework of tissue behind. As part of the healing process the skin gradually sinks down into its new shape. This helps to explain why it takes several weeks or months to see the final results of the surgery.

It is interesting to note that when liposuction was first introduced it was recommended primarily for patients under the age of 40. This was due to concern that the skin of "older"patients might not be able to redrape adequately and might, as a consequence, sag. However, this proved generally not to be the case. There are no specific age limits per se for liposuction. It is a matter of skin quality and tone, not chronological age.

In the majority of cases, the skin redrapes into a smooth contour and is essentially indistinguishable from its preoperative appearance. The skin's ability to redrape has not generally been a problem, including a liposuction performed on a 65-year-old woman. If, however, a large amount of fat is being removed from a single area, particularly if the skin is not firm, it is to be expected that the skin may not be completely taut once it redrapes. Even in extreme cases it doesn't hang (see Patient #28 for a demonstration of the skin's ability to redrape without hanging), but there may be some slight ripples or irregularities in the surface of the skin. This is more likely to occur on some parts of the body than on others. For example, the anterior thighs (the front) are more likely to have rippling postoperatively than the outer thighs. This appearance should not be confused with depressions and waves that can be seen as a result of, among other factors, extremely poor skin tone, over-resection of fat, or both. A small amount of fat removed from the stomach of an 18-year-old with firm skin tone will redrape into a flat stomach with the same skin tone under normal conditions. The removal of a large amount of fat from someone who is older will clearly result in skin tone and appearance that are less ideal than that of the 18-year-old. To a certain extent it's a trade: significantly improved overall contour but with, possibly, some slight irregularities and/or waviness. These factors should be taken into account when trying to predict the results of the surgery, and they are discussed during the consultation.

Ironically, patients who already have dimpled skin (in addition to contour irregularities), including "older" patients, may be among the best candidates for liposuction. Since they already have what could be considered an unfavorable consequence to the procedure, they have in a sense a little less at stake.

Despite this, even if the skin in its final appearance is suboptimal in comparison to the skin of a teenager, the end result is almost always a dramatic improvement and is well worth it to the patient. In many cases, the only other choices for surgical treatment of the affected areas are bigger operations (such as a tummy tuck or a thigh lift) with more noticeable scars, more risks, and much longer recovery periods than for liposuction. If it means avoiding a more significant operation, the appearance of the skin may become a secondary factor. As the photos in the case histories show, the improvements in contour are remarkable, even when the fine appearance of the skin is suboptimal.

CHAPTER 28

Who is a Candidate for Liposuction?

Anyone can undergo liposuction, but there are some people who will be more likely to benefit from the surgery than others. As with all types of cosmetic surgery, realistic expectations are an integral part of the equation.

The ideal candidate is generally considered to be someone who is at or near the ideal body weight, exercises regularly, and eats reasonably, but who has areas of contour irregularity that have been difficult to modify or eliminate. Typically, these areas are the thighs (saddle-bags), hips, and stomach for women, and the love handles, stomach, and chest for men. A near-ideal postoperative result is most likely to be achieved when patients such as these undergo liposuction. Because they are already in good shape, these people achieve excellent results with the removal of surprisingly small amounts of fat.

The most dramatic physical changes, however, are frequently seen in people who are not technically "ideal candidates." Patients who tend to be somewhat overweight but who wish to alter the contour of specific areas are often particularly satisfied with this procedure. Their body parts seem not to fit exactly right — one part, such as the upper half, is one size or shape while another, the lower half, is a different size. For these patients, buying clothing tops and bottoms in two different sizes is the norm. While total body perfection may not be anticipated, liposuction of particularly troublesome areas can provide an enormous boost in the struggle to "take control" of one's body. A liposuction of the outer thighs may enable someone to wear a straight skirt for the first time in years, likewise for a liposuction of the stomach and a narrow-waisted dress. Sometimes it's a question of dropping a size or two (or more), but sometimes it's being able to wear new types of clothes (like straight skirts) in one's current size or even just to have existing clothes fit better. The effects of the surgery are often demonstrated most strikingly in this manner.

Changes in fashion can contribute to the desire to contour specific body areas. With shorter skirts, knees are exposed; "bumps" on the inner knees often respond to liposuction. If bare midriffs or tailored waists are fashionable, then liposuction of the stomach, lower back, and/or hips may be desirable. For straight skirts, the outer thighs may be an obstacle; with sleeveless dresses the arms are more exposed and the inner arms may be the primary interest.

Finally, while true medical obesity is not amenable to correction by liposuction, even heavy patients may benefit from treatment of discrete areas that are difficult to camouflage, such as the upper arms. If liposuction is used as one component of a weight-reduction program that consists primarily of decreased caloric intake and increased activity, the results can be maximized. With significant weight loss (i.e., 100 pounds), it is likely that surgery to remove excess skin and fat, as opposed to liposuction alone, would be required. As always, the treatment for each case should be individualized.

CHAPTER 29

The Recovery

As with other surgical procedures, it's normal to have discomfort after a liposuction. The extent is unpredictable. While pain and pain perception depend on the amount of surgery, the areas treated, and the surgical technique used, they are still subject to a large degree of individual variation. The small incisions are deceptive; a lot of surgery is done through those little openings. It is normal to be sore and have discomfort in the areas of surgery for at least the first 2–3 days, after which these symptoms tend to diminish rapidly. Medication is provided to ease the discomfort, but is generally used only sparingly, particularly after the first few days. Many people describe the feeling as though one had worked out particularly hard or had fallen down. One patient commented that her recovery was easier to tolerate than having her photos taken before the surgery.

Bruising and swelling are common, although the extent is unpredictable. It is typically, but not exclusively, related to both the amount of fat removed and the technique used. Patients who tend to swell and bruise easily under normal conditions are more likely to have significant bruising post-operatively. Certain techniques (i.e., multiple incisions left open for drainage) expedite the disappearance of bruising and swelling. For the first few weeks after surgery, it is common to have scattered areas of hardness and lumps throughout the regions that were treated. In addition, tingling, numbness, and "heavy" or "funny" feelings are often reported. These symptoms disappear over several weeks or months as the healing progresses.

Activity is advanced as tolerated. This depends on the

extent of liposuction performed, as well as individual variations in recovery. Patients are encouraged to take at least a few steps the first night, and to walk about freely by the next day. Exercises, beginning slowly, may be resumed within 2–3 weeks of surgery.

The compression garment that was placed on the patient at the end of the surgery is left on, without removing it, for three days. (Cut-outs are located strategically!) For the next week, it may be removed daily for about an hour for bathing, after which it is put back on. It is worn, therefore, for a total of ten days. The garments provide compressive support, and many patients choose to wear them longer than the recommended ten days. The girdle is form-fitting and is worn easily under all but the tightest clothing; the binder typically used for stomach procedures is somewhat bulkier. With other techniques (i.e., open incisions), the garments and pads are changed frequently, starting several hours or the day after surgery. Some surgeons do not use compression garments on their patients at all.

A common concern is when one can go back to work and/or the regular routine. The answer depends, as always, on multiple factors: the amount of fat being removed, individual healing characteristics (which are difficult to predict), the type of work involved (sedentary vs. active, physical work), and the "drive" of the patient (how badly do you *want* to get back to work?). Most people can return to some form of work within a few days. If more time off can be taken, it is that much more likely that the patient will be entirely comfortable when he or she returns to work. Patients are usually examined at about 7–10 days after surgery to assess the healing, and then periodically after that. As with other types of cosmetic surgery, it is recommended that the procedure be scheduled at a time when one's social calendar is light.

CHAPTER 30

Complications of Liposuction

As with any surgical procedure, liposuction is associated with the risk of certain complications. While prevention is the key factor, early recognition and prompt treatment normally turn a potentially serious complication into a relatively minor disturbance.

Excessive bleeding, infections, blood clot formation, and inflammation of leg veins are among the complications that have been reported. With removal of more fat during a procedure than is considered safe, further problems, related to fluid shifts and blood loss, have been reported. The injection of excessive amounts of subcutaneous fluid can be associated with toxic levels of lidocaine and/or epinephrine. Other, usually temporary, conditions, such as swelling, bruising, and changes in pigmentation and sensation of the legs (numbness, tingling), are actually expected to occur and are not truly considered to be complications. Small seromas may form, particularly if large amounts of fluid were injected subcutaneously and/or if drainage was suboptimal. Many other complications have been reported although they are rare.

Contour irregularities are generally considered unfavorable results, rather than complications. Suboptimal postoperative contours are essentially due either to too much fat remaining or too little fat remaining. Occasionally, both situations are seen simultaneously in different areas of the same patient. As has been previously explained, the final result of a liposuction depends not only on the amount and distribution of the fat removed at the time of surgery, but on the skin's ability to redrape itself to the new contour. If indicated, additional fat can be removed several months after the surgery. The recovery for a secondary procedure is, in general, easier than for a primary procedure. While the explanation for this is unclear, it is probably because a much smaller amount of fat is usually removed at a secondary procedure, and because internal adhesions (scar tissue from the first procedure) limit the amount of swelling that typically occurs. Excess scar tissue, which may form as part of the healing process, can also be treated the same way.

It is easier to treat a patient who has too much fat remaining than someone who has too little fat remaining. For this reason, it is important that the fat resection be conservative at the initial procedure. While the goal is a single, perfect procedure, the need to remove some additional fat from one or more areas is a relatively minimal concern, aside from the inconvenience to the patient. It indicates that the first procedure was somewhat more cautious than was necessary.

The treatment of a depressed area is, understandably, more difficult. In general, a combination of further sculpting ("feathering") of the edges of the depressions and adding some filling material (such as a series of fat transplants from other areas of the body) is used. In most cases, these areas can be significantly improved in this manner even if not corrected completely; that depends, at least partly, on the extent of the problem.

CHAPTER 31

Can You Have More Done if You Want To?

For a variety of reasons, many of which are noted above, there are times when a patient who has had this procedure wishes to undergo more liposuction. This may be to recontour new areas, to do more in areas that were already treated, or both. If new areas are to be done, it is the same as undergoing the procedure for the first time. Doing more in areas that have already been treated is often referred to as a "secondary," "touch-up," or "revision" liposuction. This is normally a relatively minor procedure. Sometimes one or two areas are involved, sometimes multiple areas. The specific indications for this surgery depend on the physical appearance of the areas before and after surgery, the expectations of the patient, the individual healing character-istics of the patient, and other factors such as subsequent weight gain or loss, change in exercise pattern, etc. With a secondary liposuction, there is normally a shorter operative time, a faster recovery (less bruising, swelling, and discomfort), and a decreased need for postoperative compression when compared with the primary procedure. Minor seroma formation postoper-atively may be somewhat more likely with a secondary procedure. This is due to characteristics of the internal scar tissue left by the first procedure. Local anesthesia, possibly with light sedation, is often adequate even if the original procedure was performed using deeper sedation. Typically, a weekend is enough recovery time. In general, existing incisions can be used; in some cases, one or more additional incisions are required. The same principles of small, hidden incisions and scars that are used for primary liposuction apply to revision procedures as well.

CHAPTER 32

Ultrasonic Liposuction (Ultrasonic Assisted Lipoplasty)

Ultrasonic liposuction represents the latest technological development in lipoplasty. It uses a new method to remove fat. Instead of the fat being removed mechanically (with the cannulas and suction machine of traditional liposuction), ultrasonic waves are used to "melt" the fat, after which the liquid remnants are suctioned out.

This procedure is performed in the following manner: (1) several incisions are made in the skin, (2) a large amount of fluid is injected subcutaneously, (3) specialized probes are inserted into the fat, (4) ultrasonic waves generated by a machine melt the fat (actually, they break up the fat cells, producing a soupy mix of fat cell remnants), (5) the resultant liquid is aspirated,[22] and (6) traditional liposuction is used to contour further the regions being treated, as well as to taper and contour the edges around those areas.

Proponents of ultrasonic liposuction cite the following advantages of this technique versus traditional liposuction:

First, because the technology preferentially melts the fat (before affecting the other structures, e.g., blood vessels and nerves), large amounts of fat can be removed while producing somewhat less blood loss. This makes ultrasonic liposuction particularly advantageous for large volume resections of fat. As stated above, however, much less blood loss has been reported with the superwet and tumescent techniques of liposuction than with preinjecting less vasoconstricting fluid. Therefore, this aspect of ultrasonic liposuction is less of an advantage than it would have been previously. Furthermore,

---

[22] Newer hollow cannulas combine melting and some of the aspiration into one instrument.

for safety considerations many plastic surgeons prefer not to do large volume resections at a single time, opting instead to treat these patients with two or more procedures.

A second beneficial property of ultrasonic liposuction is its apparent ability to help skin retract, or tighten, postoperatively. This can be particularly useful when there is a large amount of excess or loose skin, whether existing or anticipated as a result of the procedure. While the explanation for this is not certain, it is presumably a consequence of the energy generated by this technique.

A third advantage is that the ultrasonic technique seems to "ferret" out fat from areas that are harder to treat with traditional liposuction, i.e., where there is relatively more thick, fibrous tissue than in other areas. These include the back and upper stomach (above the belly button), and the male breast. These areas can be treated effectively with traditional liposuction although the surgeon has to work somewhat harder in order to do so adequately.

A fourth advantage is that the ultrasonic technique is less strenuous on the surgeon. This is because it melts the fat; this difference is particularly significant when contouring the areas noted above. Since the ultrasonic probe does most of the work, there is less stress on the surgeon's arm. Fat can be removed more easily when using the ultrasonic technique.

Fluid is injected subcutaneously for two reasons. First, the ultrasonic procedure generates heat as the fat is being melted.[23] The surrounding tissues must be cooled with a constant infusion of chilled fluid in order to prevent a thermal injury, i.e., a burn. Full thickness burns of the skin, extending outward from the deep subcutaneous tissues, have been reported when inadequate cooling was used and/or when the probe was too close to the skin. This is enough of a concern so that ultrasonic liposuction is not generally recommended for use on thin regions like the face and neck, inner thighs, and inner knees, as well as any areas where there is relatively little fat. Second, as with traditional liposuction, the fluid provides

---

[23] Newer designs incorporate a self-cooling mechanism, although it is not yet clear that this problem has been eliminated.

both vasoconstriction and perioperative pain relief.

There are several disadvantages of ultrasonic liposuction at present. Traditional liposuction cannulas can be curved, bent, and adapted as needed to reach multiple areas from each incision. Ultrasonic probes are more fragile and cannot be bent. In fact, the machine automatically pauses when too much torque is produced. Furthermore, the probes (and the accessories required for their use) are thicker than traditional liposuction cannulas so that larger incisions are required.

The ultrasonic probe treats not only the area at the immediate tip, but also a surrounding zone of several millimeters (an eighth of an inch or so). A wider area of contouring is thus accomplished when working from a single incision. For surgeons who normally use multiple incisions with traditional liposuction, the fewer incisions used with ultrasonic constitute an advantage. Surgeons who already use fewer incisions, however, feel that the larger and more evident incisions necessitated by the ultrasonic technique are a distinct disadvantage. This is even more true if, as is often the case, they must be placed in more visible locations. Thus, the incisions required for ultrasonic liposuction are relatively larger and in more visible locations; depending on how the traditional liposuction is done, they may be more numerous as well.

Early reports suggested that there is less pain postoperatively among patients who had ultrasonic liposuction as part of their procedure. This has not truly been borne out with time, although it appears to be true for the first few days. Some surgeons have noted more and/or different postoperative pain among these patients, some note less pain, and others have reported no noticeable difference between the two techniques.

Incorporating the ultrasonic technique often prolongs the operating time and, therefore, the anesthesia. This is because after the ultrasonic liposuction has been done, it is necessary to use traditional liposuction to contour and feather the edges, which would otherwise be associated with a higher risk of burns because the areas are thinner.

Finally, as noted above, the heat generated by the ultrasonic technique can be a problem. Instances of burned areas, including skin surrounding the incision, underlying tissue, and wide areas overlying the regions being treated, have been reported. Some of these burns have been significant, necessitating treatment typically used for patients who have sustained severe thermal (e.g., fire) or chemical (e.g., acid) burns. The heat generated may also be responsible for another less serious though troublesome complication that has been reported — an increased risk of seroma formation (when compared with traditional liposuction). Seromas, which are collections of straw-colored fluid beneath the skin, are known consequences of abdominoplasties (tummy tucks) and can also occur with liposuction. If accurate, their reported increased incidence with the ultrasonic technique may be due as much to the large amount of fluid used as to the technique itself.

As of this writing, the full potential impact of this technology is not clear.[24] While the development of thinner cannulas will allow smaller incisions, it seems less likely that surgeons will be able to use the fewer distant, hidden incisions that can be used with traditional liposuction. Ultrasonic liposuction will continue to have a place in plastic surgery; the question is exactly what that is. Some surgeons use it on the majority of their liposuctions. Many use it selectively, adding this "tool" to their "tool belt." The extent to which it is used may depend on the surgeon's preference as well as the type of patients he or she typically sees. For many reasons, some surgeons' practices are composed primarily of patients who are relatively thin and who need less contouring, and others' of patients who are relatively large and who undergo larger removals of fat. The ultrasonic technique appears to be particularly useful for large volume reductions, and when relatively larger and/or more visible scars are acceptable. Despite its intriguing technology, the benefits of this procedure for the average patient remain

---

[24] The latest use of ultrasonic technology is to apply it externally (i.e., directly onto the skin) prior to using traditional liposuction. Despite claims that this combination works better that liposuction alone, the use of external ultrasound has not yet been validated by scientific studies.

debatable. The potential problems of scars that are more numerous, more visible, and larger, and a longer operating time are discussed above. It can be argued that the need to use larger and more visible scars (and often more numerous) is enough of a reason not to select ultrasonic liposuction for most patients. Its ultimate role remains, at this point, a topic of speculation.

CHAPTER 33

Liposuction for Men

Cosmetic surgery among men represents one of the fastest growing segments. Liposuction for men is similar to the procedure for women, and most of what is written above applies to men as well. In general, however, different areas are treated.

The most common areas treated are the neck, the love handles (with or without the rest of the stomach), and the chest (male breasts or "gynecomastia"). These areas accumulate fat preferentially in men. Expanding waistlines often propel men to undergo liposuction. Pants that once fit comfortably may start to cause mild discomfort or may ride a bit lower each year.

Men are more likely than women to have fat in areas that are not accessible to liposuction, i.e., deep to one or more muscles. In the neck, the fat may be deep to the platysma muscle (the thin muscle of the neck that is tensed while shaving); in the stomach, it may be deep to the abdominal wall (i.e., around the intestines). In the first case, it is only minimally accessible by liposuction; in the second, not at all. As in other cases, the relative distribution and proportions of fat above and below the muscle are assessed during the consultation. The likelihood of success with liposuction can be estimated at this time.

Just as the stomach, hips, and thighs are often treated together in women, the chest, stomach, and love handles are often treated together in men. The reason is the same: to maintain balance and ensure that any postoperative weight gain will leave the body remaining proportionate. When a significant liposuction is performed on the stomach and love handles (the most commonly requested areas), the chest may become more noticeable postoperatively, particularly if there is any weight gain. Treating all three areas together maintains desirable proportions.

As in women, the male breast consists of both fat and breast tissue. Male breast tissue tends to be extremely dense. Liposuction is most effective on fat, so the more fat that is present, the easier the contouring is likely to be. Nevertheless, most enlarged breasts can be treated with liposuction alone. Occasionally, direct excision of breast tissue is required, using an incision around the lower portion of the nipple. If a significant excess of skin is present, a procedure that removes that excess and tightens the remaining skin may be necessary.

Men have somewhat of an advantage when it comes to the skin. From an anatomical standpoint, their skin (including deeper, subcutaneous tissues) is thicker and denser than that of women. The thickness of these tissues provides a buffer and helps mask potential contour irregularities resulting from the surgery. Skin and subcutaneous tissue thickness varies, both between individuals and on different parts of the same person. As with women, incisions are hidden where possible. For men, this means they are placed in natural creases or within hair-bearing areas. Depending on the hair pattern, camouflaging the incisions may be more or less difficult.

The denser subcutaneous tissue makes the procedure more difficult technically from the surgeon's standpoint, and because this tissue has more blood vessels than fat, there may be somewhat more bleeding. While ultrasonic liposuction appears to have an advantage in removing fat in these areas, it also generates more heat. Denser tissues accumulate and retain heat more than looser, fatty tissues do, thereby increasing the risk of a burn. Regardless of the technique used, the increased thickness of the tissues means that noticeable contour irregularities are less likely in men than in women, helping to make men excellent candidates for liposuction.

Section 4
Tummy Tucks and Mini-Tummy Tucks

CHAPTER 34

Tummy Tucks and Mini-Tummy Tucks

An abdominoplasty, also called a tummy tuck, removes excess skin and fat from the stomach. It is, conceptually, a relatively simple procedure. A horizontal (transverse) incision is made near the lower portion of the abdomen, usually just above the pubic hair. The incision (and the resulting scar) extends across the front of the lower abdomen, nearly from one hip bone to the other. In most cases, it is either gently curved or W-shaped, with rounded points. The scar this procedure leaves, coupled with the development and domination of liposuction and modified abdominal procedures, has decreased its popularity. Nevertheless, there are many cases in which it is the best option; sometimes it's the only one. Once the incision is made, the skin is separated from the muscles underneath (the "abs"). Starting from that point, the skin is lifted up as far as the ribs (an incision is made around the belly button, which is left in place). The abdominal skin is then stretched and pulled down, the excess is removed, and the skin is sewn back together. An incision is made in the skin and the belly button is brought through and sewn into place so that the patient keeps her own belly button; i.e., a new hole for the old belly button. In most cases, all of the skin between the belly button and the lower incision can be removed. The muscles of the abdomen (or more precisely the connective tissue covering them) are usually tightened as part of this procedure. Many different variations of this procedure, in terms of precise location and pattern of the incisions, as well as additional minor procedures and maneuvers that can be performed to tighten the connective tissues further, are in use. The basics of the operation, however, are the removal of excess skin and, if indicated, the tightening of the abdominal muscles.

An increasingly popular variant of this procedure is called a mini-abdominoplasty or mini-tummy tuck. This procedure combines liposuction of the stomach with the removal of some skin from the lower abdomen. It is designed for patients who have excess skin and fat below the belly button, but relatively taut skin, with or without some excess fat, above it. This procedure starts with a liposuction of the entire stomach (abdomen), as needed. Next, a horizontal incision (up to about half the length of the full tummy tuck) is made in approximately the same location as described above. Again, the skin is separated from the underlying muscles and is lifted up in the direction of the umbilicus. In this case, however, the dissection stops there. The muscles of the lower abdomen are tightened, the excess skin is removed, and the incision is closed.

Patients who already have scars on their lower abdomen are particularly good candidates for this procedure. Scars resulting from Caesarean sections and ovarian or uterine surgery may be located in or near the location of the incision used for this procedure. When present, these scars can often be used, sometimes requiring a slight extension, for a mini-tummy tuck. A mini-tummy tuck is most effective when the protrusion of the lower abdomen (below the navel) is due primarily to excess skin, with or without excess fat, rather than to muscle or abdominal wall weakness, in which case a full tummy tuck may be indicated.

Selecting the appropriate procedure (tummy tuck, mini-tummy tuck, or liposuction alone) depends on the anatomy of the person in question. As always, it is important to determine which anatomical features are responsible for one's appearance. The initial exam of the abdomen is performed by tensing the stomach muscles and feeling what's on top. Components can include excess skin, excess fat, a combination of the two, weakness of the abdominal muscles, or any of a variety of internal abdominal problems. Weakness or separation of the abdominal muscles (the "abs") is common, particularly among women who have had relatively large babies, multiple pregnancies, and/or twins. Findings can be different in different parts of the abdomen. These factors need to be assessed, occasionally requiring the input of another doctor, such as a general surgeon.

Sometimes the preferred treatment is obvious. In cases of massive weight loss (such as more than 100 pounds, or a certain percentage of one's body weight), there is often a clear excess of skin, and removal of that skin is the only procedure that will improve the appearance. Significant weight loss may also warrant skin removal in other regions, such as the breasts, arms, thighs, and back. Some variants of these procedures can be more extensive than a standard tummy tuck. A procedure called a Lower Body Lift elevates and tightens the skin of the abdomen, hips, and thighs. It leaves a scar that extends completely around the body at the level of the lower abdomen, and it is more involved (longer hospitalization, possible blood transfusions, etc.) than the procedures described in this book, but in all fairness, it accomplishes things that they do not.

The presence of certain medical conditions may preclude these procedures (primarily the full tummy tuck) from being performed safely. This is because the blood supply to the skin is a particular concern with tummy tucks. Skin and tissues normally receive their blood supply from vessels that run both horizontally (i.e., within the skin) and vertically (i.e., come up from deeper tissues). When the skin is lifted up, the vertical blood vessels are cut, so it must survive based solely on the network that runs within the skin. Skin elevated in this manner is referred to as a "flap." Anything that affects the circulation of the flap increases the risk of complications. Medical conditions that may do this include diabetes and autoimmune diseases, such as lupus erythematosus, Raynaud's disease, and scleroderma, all of which are characterized by narrowing and decreased function of the small blood vessels on which such flaps are dependent. Heart and kidney conditions may have similar effects. This also explains why it may not be safe to perform a liposuction of the upper portion of the abdomen at the same time as a tummy tuck. The trauma of this procedure, with its resultant swelling and compression of blood vessels, can impair the blood supply to the lower portion of the skin. Two procedures, at different times, may be required to achieve optimal results in these patients. For example, after a tummy tuck is performed to reduce the excess skin, a liposuction may be needed several months later to recontour the fat. Liposuction of other portions of the body, such as the hips and thighs, can usually be performed safely at the same time as the tummy tuck. This concern with blood supply does not normally apply to mini-tummy tucks, and liposuction can usually be done to multiple areas, including the upper abdomen, at the same time as this procedure.

Tobacco use (i.e., smoking) is among the non-medical conditions that can have the same effects on tummy tucks (as well as facelifts, which also depend on flaps that require healthy small blood vessels). Studies have confirmed the effect of tobacco smoking on small blood vessels. It has not been determined whether stopping smoking for a specific period of time before and/or after the surgery decreases the risks associated with it, but it certainly seems prudent to do so. The presence of scars on the abdomen can also affect the planning for this procedure. Normal blood flow may be disrupted by scars. Although tissues that have been cut will heal, the blood vessels (as well as nerves and other tissues) do not immediately, if ever, return to their complete preoperative anatomy. The presence of certain scars, depending on their location, orientation, and size, may preclude doing a tummy tuck safely.

CHAPTER 35

Complications of Tummy Tucks

Complications that can occur as a result of this surgery include some that are specific for tummy tucks, in addition to those discussed above. As with other procedures, one or more areas of the stomach may have altered sensation after the surgery. Much of this is temporary, although it can take up to a year or more to resolve. Normally sensation is diminished (i.e., areas are numb); sometimes there is tingling or a heavy feeling. Some of the altered sensation may be permanent.

The appearance of the scar is another potential issue. The horizontal scar is an integral and unavoidable part of this procedure. Ideally, the incision heals into a relatively unobtrusive scar, but as noted above, scars are somewhat unpredictable. Furthermore, in order to achieve the maximum cosmetic result, the abdominal tissues must be closed under a certain amount of tension; otherwise, the skin may be too loose, which partially defeats the purpose of the procedure. Excess tension increases the possibility of a less desirable scar. During the surgery, deep sutures are inserted to remove some of the tension from the skin itself. If, despite this, the scar heals in an unfavorable manner, it can often be treated with injections of an anti-inflammatory substance, a scar revision (a procedure that improves the appearance of a scar), or a combination of the two.

Another complication is seroma formation. A seroma is a collection of straw-colored fluid that accumulates under the healing skin before the repositioned skin of the stomach adheres sufficiently to the abdominal wall. This fluid is similar to the fluid that oozes out from a scraped knee. Tubes (called "drains") that draw out fluid are routinely placed under the skin at the end of the procedure to prevent this from happening; these evacuate the fluid that typically accumulates during the first few days after the surgery. They are normally left in place for up to a week, after which they are removed during an office visit. A seroma can form if the fluid is inadequately drained and/or continues to accumulate after the drains are removed.

When seromas do occur, they are treated initially with aspiration (using a fine needle to withdraw the fluid), reinsertion of one or more drains, or a combination. When identified and treated early, this complication is usually transient and produces only minimal disturbance. If allowed to persist, or rarely, for unexplained reasons in spite of early intervention, a second surgical procedure is required to expedite the adherence of the skin to the abdominal wall.

Early movement and ambulation (i.e., getting up out of bed, sitting, and walking around) has markedly diminished the likelihood of developing blood clots in the legs, which was once a major risk of this surgery. The most significant local complication is delayed wound and skin healing which, at its extreme, leads to thicker scars. Excessive bleeding, infection, and conditions that reduce blood flow, such as diabetes, circulatory disorders, and tobacco use, predispose to this complication, as do excess tension of the skin closure and early overexertion. As with all complications, it is not always possible to identify precisely why any specific one has occurred.

Section 5
Results

The following is photographic documentation of the types of results that can be achieved with plastic surgery. The cases were chosen because they demonstrate the effects of specific procedures. Not all patients can get all results; each postoperative result should be judged in comparison with the preoperative anatomy, rather than by an absolute standard.

The "after" photos were taken at least three months following the surgical procedures. Every attempt was made to standardize the preoperative and postoperative photos in terms of distance, angle, exposure, lighting, makeup, etc. In one case potentially identifying jewelry was "erased;" aside from this, no photos were retouched or altered. The effects of surgery can be enhanced, and nearly duplicated, by manipulating some or all of these factors. This has been shown repeatedly and is seen in many "makeovers."[25]

Signed releases were obtained from all patients whose photos appear in this book.

---

[25] Becker, H. The computer and truth. *Plast. Reconstr. Surg.* 94: 896, 1994.

CHAPTER 36

Breast Enlargements

The choices of implant location (above or below the muscle) and the three incisions used most commonly for breast enlargement are shown in Figures #1 and #2, respectively. The incisions are the axillary (under the arm), periareolar (around the areola, the dark area surrounding the nipple), and the inframammary (under the breast). A fourth, the umbilical, is used only rarely. Once the scars fade, it is normally not possible to tell from the photographs which approach was used. It is similarly difficult to tell whether the implants are above or below the pectoral muscle, or what type of implants they are. The age of each patient, the approach (incision) used, and the type and position of the implant used are indicated. Also shown in this section are the correction of tuberous breasts and breast enlargement with a lift. Both procedures use breast implants in addition to other techniques.

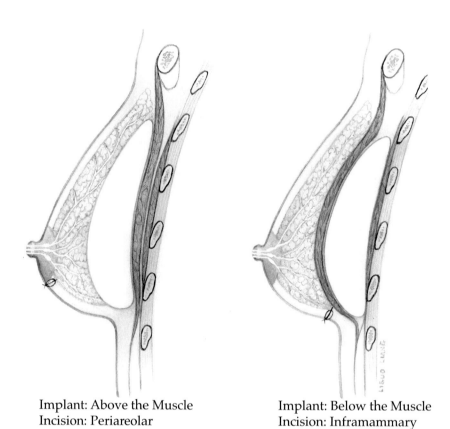

Implant: Above the Muscle
Incision: Periareolar

Implant: Below the Muscle
Incision: Inframammary

Figure 1. Breast Implants: Above / Below the Muscle

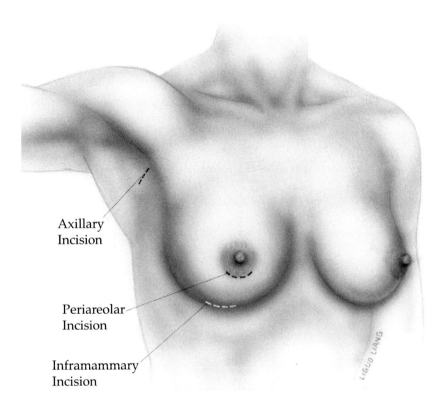

Axillary
Incision

Periareolar
Incision

Inframammary
Incision

Figure 2. Breast Implant Incisions

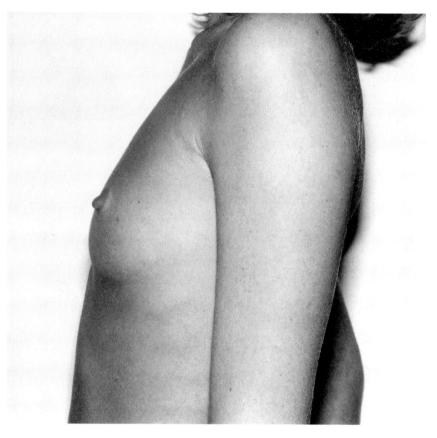

Patient Number:	*1*
Age, etc.:	28 years old, 5'9" tall, 115 lbs
Implant:	160 cc, Round, Textured Silicone
Location/Incision:	Above Muscle / Inframammary
Bra size:	34 A (Pre-Op) ---> 34 B (Post-Op)

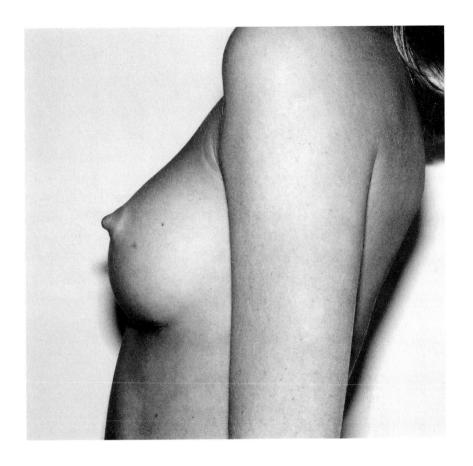

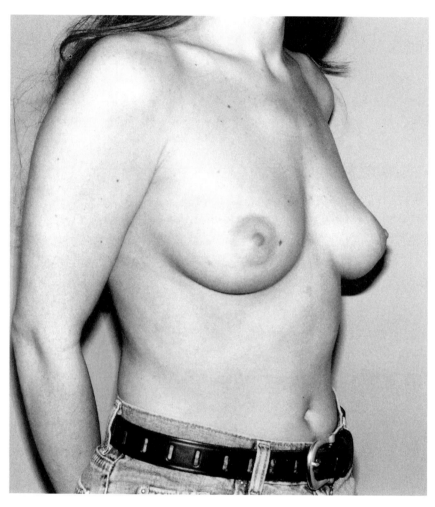

Patient Number: 2
Age, etc.:   27 years old, 5'2" tall, 115 lbs
Implant: 225 cc, Round, Smooth Saline
Location/Incision: Below Muscle / Periareolar
Bra size: 34 B (Pre-Op) ---> 34 Full C (Post-Op)

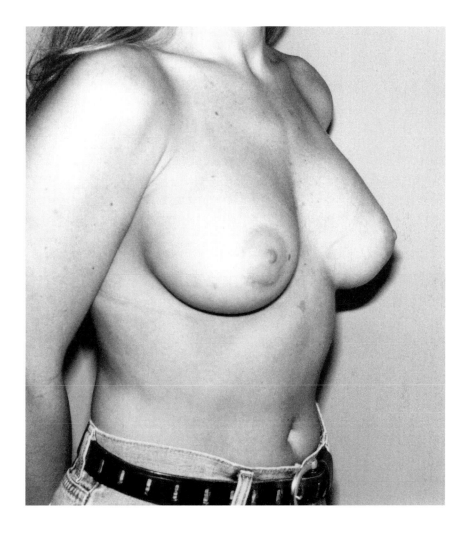

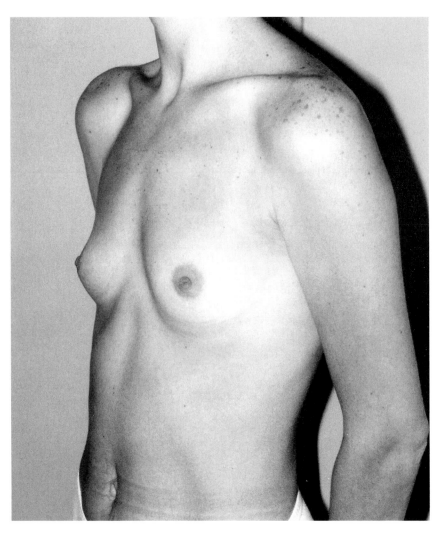

Patient Number: 3
Age, etc.:   27 years old, 5'7" tall, 115 lbs
Implant: 325 cc, Round, Textured Saline
Location/Incision: Below Muscle / Periareolar
Bra size: 34 AA (Pre-Op) ---> 34 C (Post-Op)

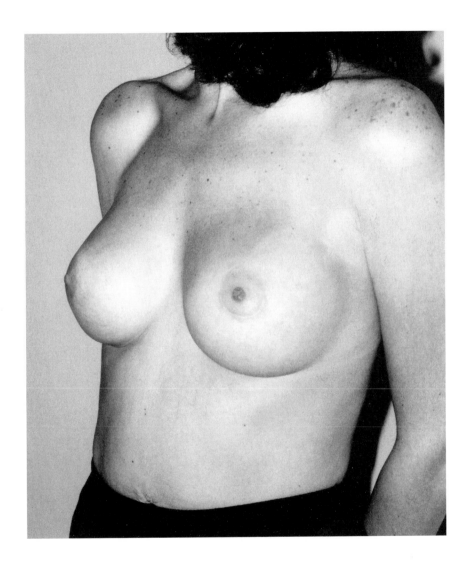

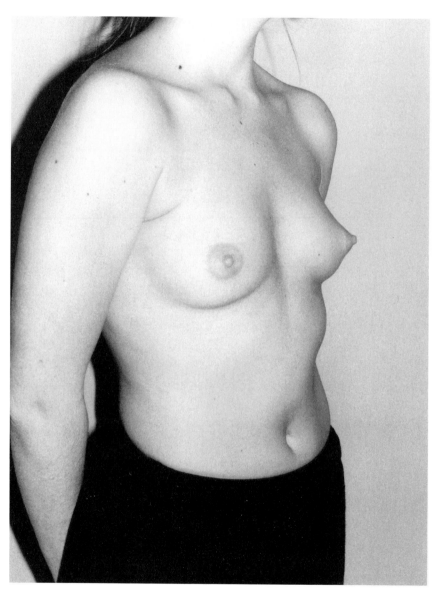

Patient Number:	*4*
Age, etc.:	18 years old, 5'2" tall, 110 lbs
Implant:	300 cc, Round, Smooth Saline
Location/Incision:	Below Muscle / Periareolar
Bra size:	34 A (Pre-Op) ---> 34 C (Post-Op)

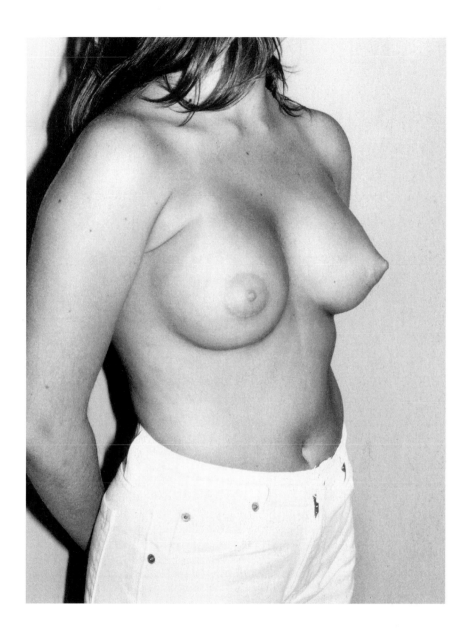

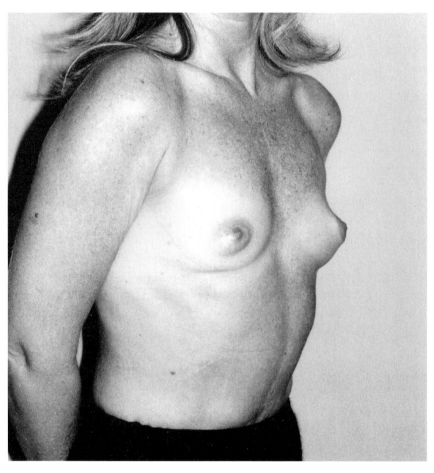

Patient Number: 5
Age, etc.:   37 years old, 5'5" tall, 125 lbs
Implant: 225 cc, Round, Smooth Saline
Location/Incision: Below Muscle / Periareolar
Bra size: 34 A (Pre-Op) ---> 34 B (Post-Op)

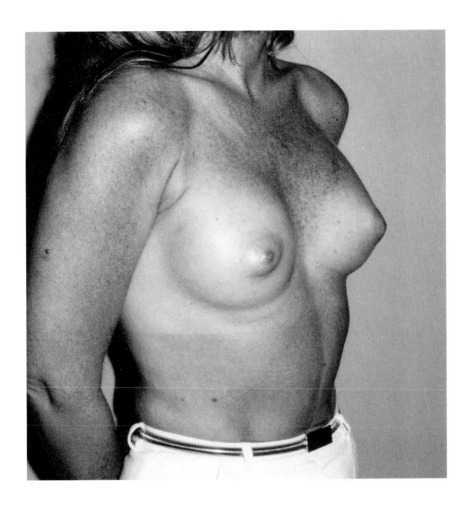

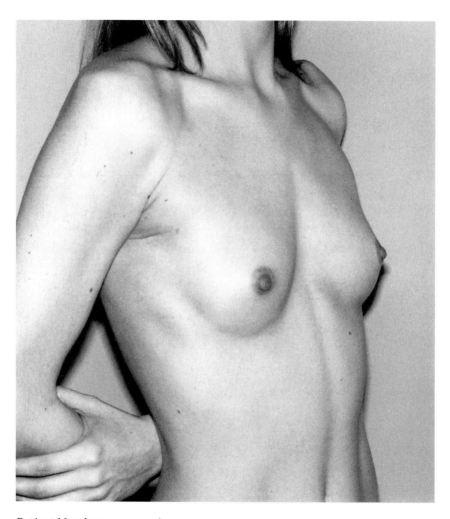

Patient Number:	6
Age, etc.:	27 years old, 5'10 1/2" tall, 130 lbs
Implant:	325 cc, Round, Textured Saline
Location/Incision:	Below Muscle / Periareolar
Bra size:	34 A (Pre-Op) ---> 34 C (Post-Op)

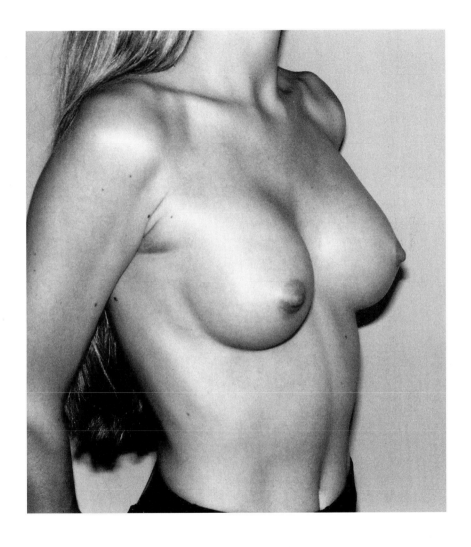

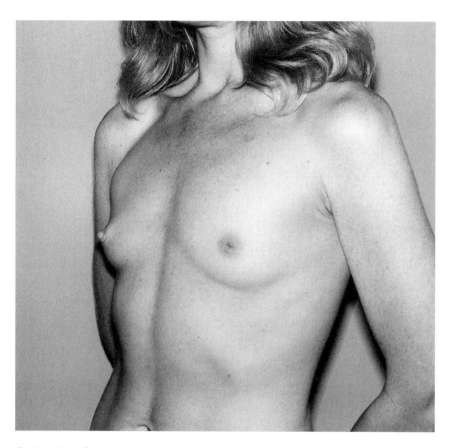

Patient Number: 7
Age, etc.:   36 years old, 5'8" tall, 130 lbs
Implant: 375 cc, Round, Smooth Saline
Location/Incision: Below Muscle / Periareolar
Bra size: 34 A (Pre-Op) ---> 34 Full C (Post-Op)

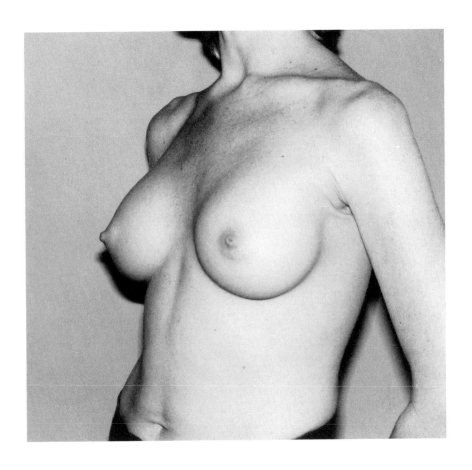

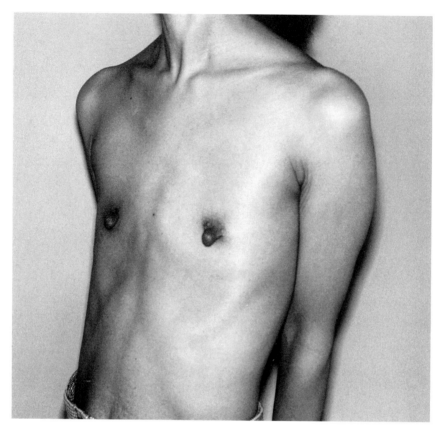

Patient Number:	8
Age, etc.:	35 years old, 5'3" tall, 90 lbs
Implant:	250 cc, Round, Smooth Saline
Location/Incision:	Below Muscle / Axillary
Bra size:	34 No Cup (Pre-Op) ---> 34 B (Post-Op)

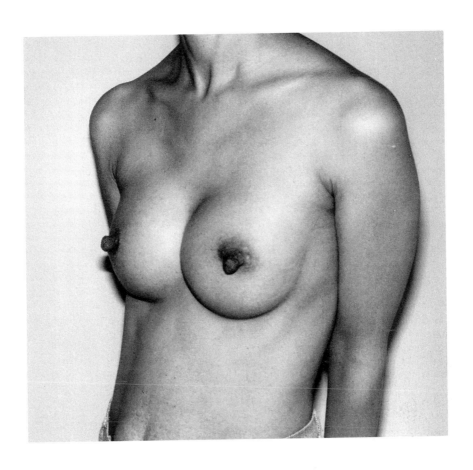

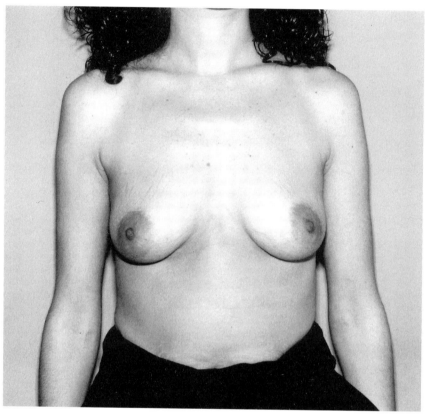

Patient Number:	*9*
Age, etc.:	30 years old, 5'0" tall, 101 lbs
Implant:	275 cc, Round, Textured Saline
Location/Incision:	Below Muscle / Periareolar
Bra size:	34 B (Pre-Op) ---> 34 D (Post-Op)

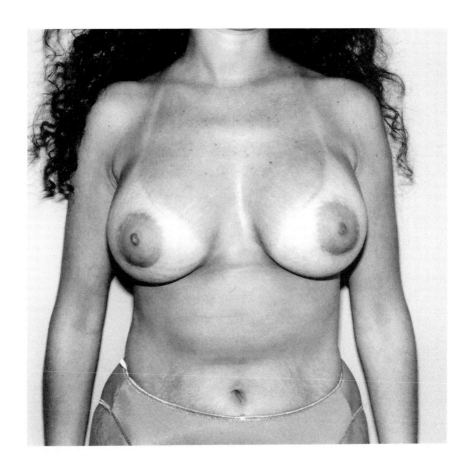

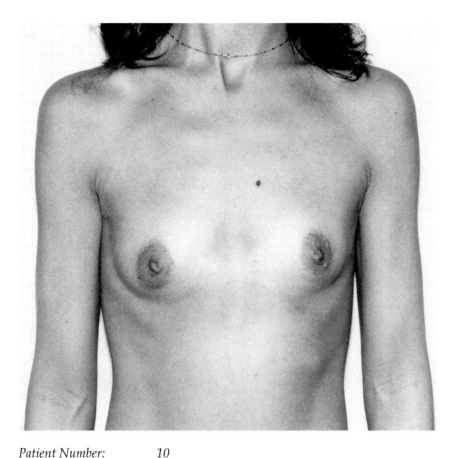

Patient Number:	*10*
Age, etc.:	34 years old, 5'7" tall, 120 lbs
Implant:	275 cc, Round, Textured Saline
Location/Incision:	Above Muscle / Periareolar
Bra size:	34 AA (Pre-Op) ---> 34 B (Post-Op)

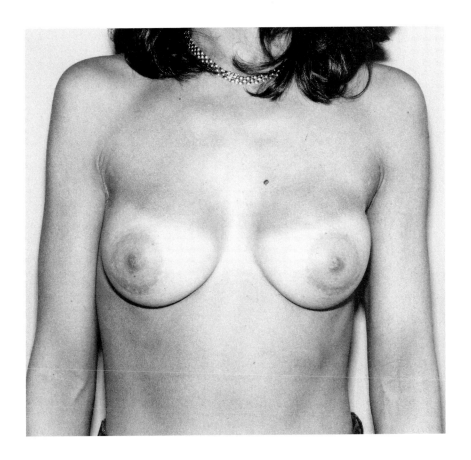

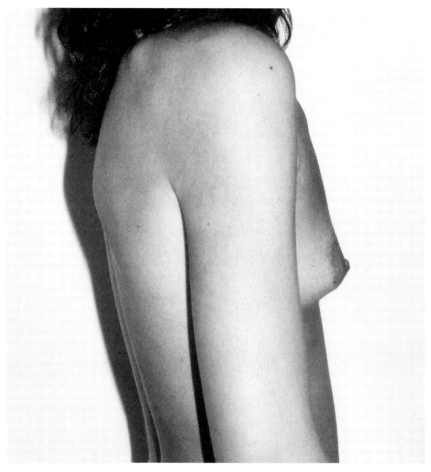

Patient Number:	*10 (cont.)*
Age, etc.:	34 years old, 5'7" tall, 120 lbs
Implant:	275 cc, Round, Textured Saline
Location/Incision:	Above Muscle / Periareolar
Bra size:	34 AA (Pre-Op) ---> 34 B (Post-Op)

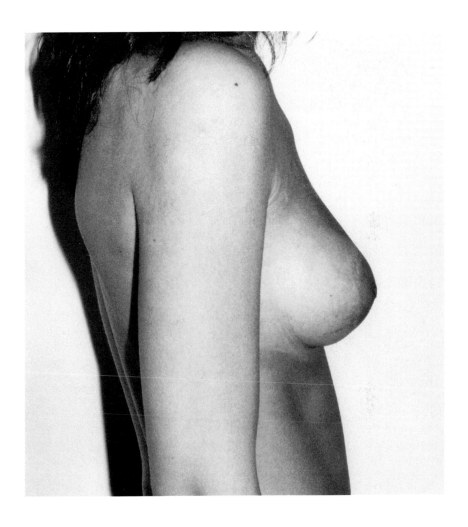

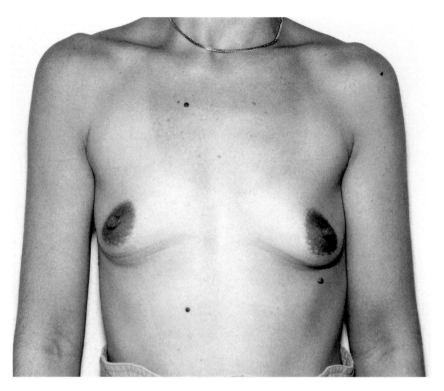

Patient Number:	*11*
Age, etc.:	34 years old, 5'4" tall, 122 lbs
Implant:	250 cc, Round, Textured Silicone
Location/Incision:	Above Muscle / Periareolar
Bra size:	34 AA (Pre-Op) ---> 34 B (Post-Op)

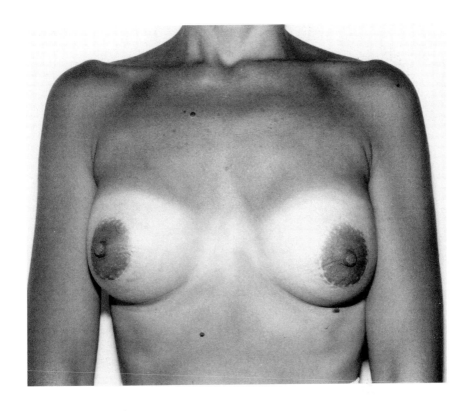

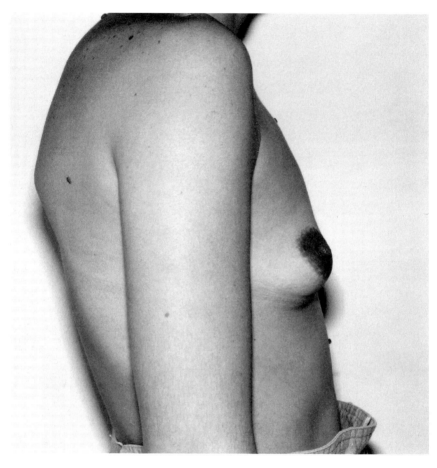

Patient Number:	*11 (cont.)*
Age, etc.:	34 years old, 5'4" tall, 122 lbs
Implant:	250 cc, Round, Textured Silicone
Location / Incision:	Above Muscle / Periareolar
Bra size:	34 AA (Pre-Op) ---> 34 B (Post-Op)

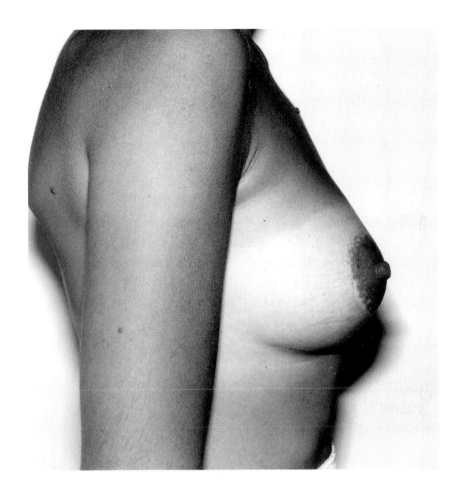

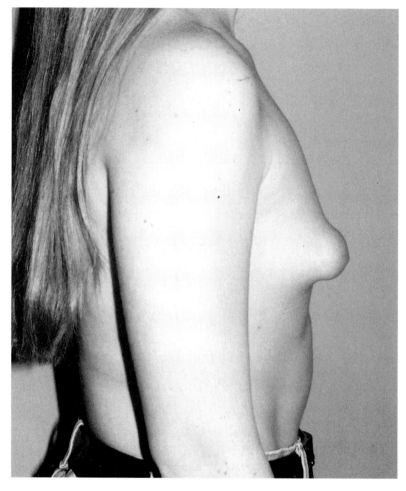

Patient Number:	*12 (Correction of Tuberous Breasts)*
Age, etc.:	20 years old, 5'4" tall, 120 lbs
Implant:	275 cc, Round, Textured Saline
Location/Incision:	Below Muscle / Periareolar
Bra size:	34 AA (Pre-Op) ---> 34 B (Post-Op)

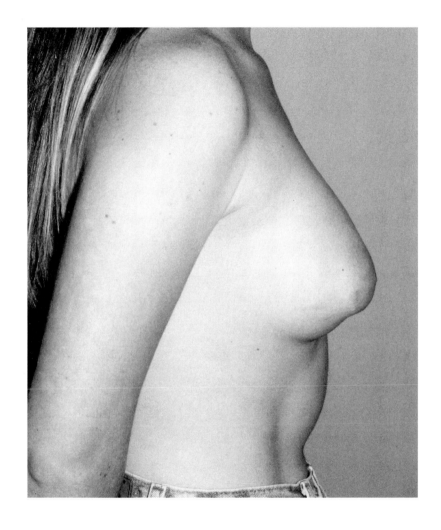

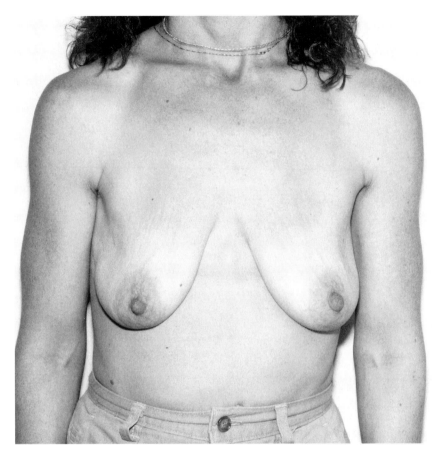

Patient Number:	*13 (Breast Lift with Implants)*
Age, etc.:	41 years old, 5'2" tall, 118 lbs
Implant:	240 cc, Round, Textured Saline
Location/Incision:	Above Muscle / Anchor-shaped
Bra size:	34 A (Pre-Op) ---> 34 C (Post-Op)

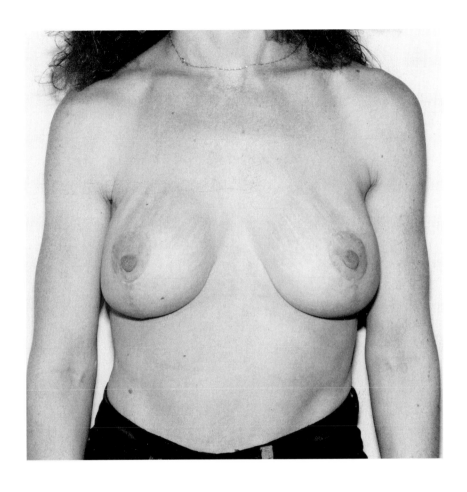

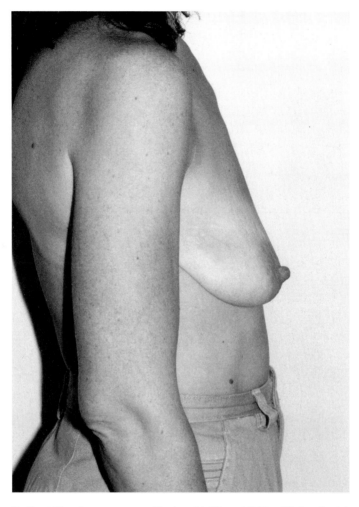

Patient Number: 13 *(cont.) (Breast Lift with Implants)*
Age, etc.:   41 years old, 5'2" tall, 118 lbs
Implant: 240 cc, Round, Textured Saline
Location/Incision: Above Muscle / Anchor-shaped
Bra size: 34 A (Pre-Op) ---> 34 C (Post-Op)

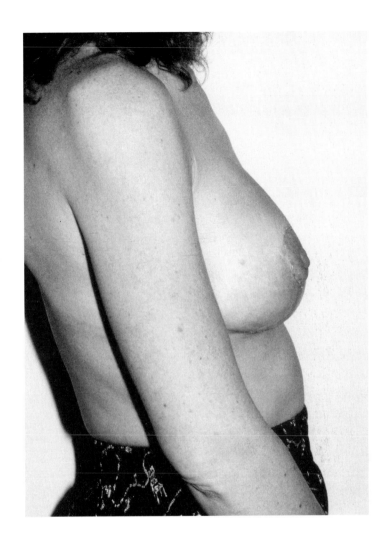

CHAPTER 37

Breast Lifts and Reductions

Since breast lifts and reductions are similar operations, the patients shown here exhibit similar scar patterns. The incisions for the vertical mammaplasty and the anchor-shaped reduction are shown in Figure #3. These are visible to different degrees, depending largely on individual variations in healing. The size of the breasts postoperatively is based on the preoperative size and the preferences of the patient. Not all postoperative sizes can be made aesthetically from all preoperative sizes; excess removal of breast tissue may preclude recreating the conical shape that is generally desired. For example, if a patient with a double *D* cup size wanted to be an *A*, the resultant shape of the breast (even assuming that could be done) would be too flat and wide. Another reason to limit the extent of the reduction is to keep the breast size reasonably proportionate to the rest of the body. Candidates for breast reduction often have relatively broad shoulders and torsos; very small breasts may look peculiar on these women. The first case is a breast lift; the remainder are breast reductions.

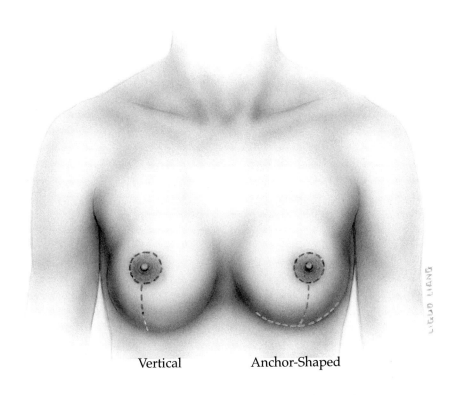

Vertical   Anchor-Shaped

Figure 3. Breast Lift / Reduction Incisions

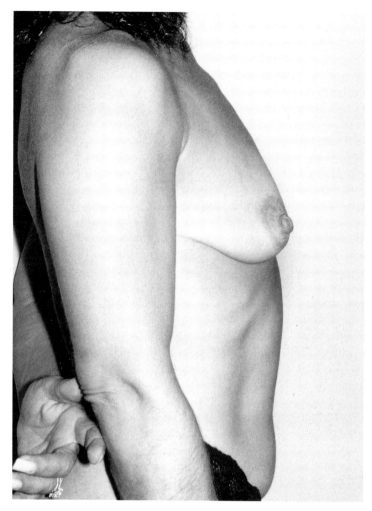

Patient Number:	*14*
Age:	45 years old
Incision Pattern:	Vertical

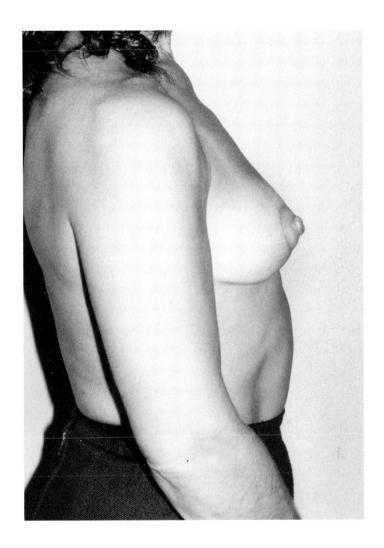

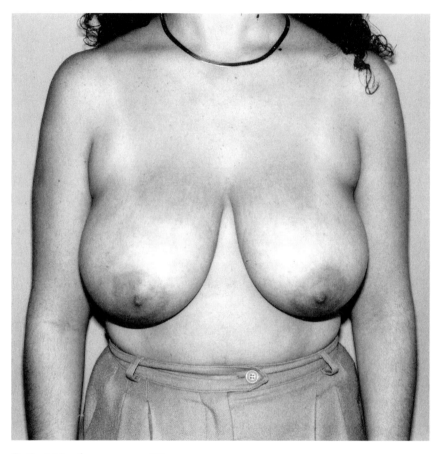

Patient Number :	*15*
Age:	28 years old
Incision Pattern:	Vertical

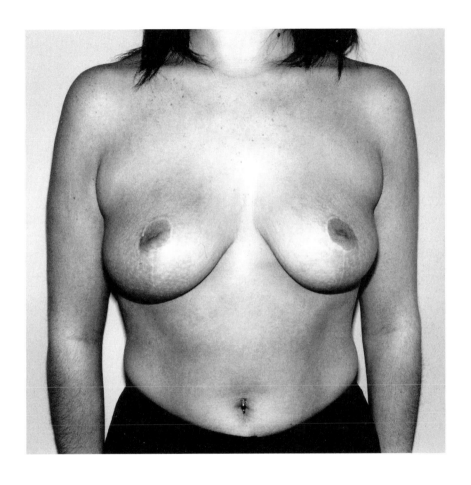

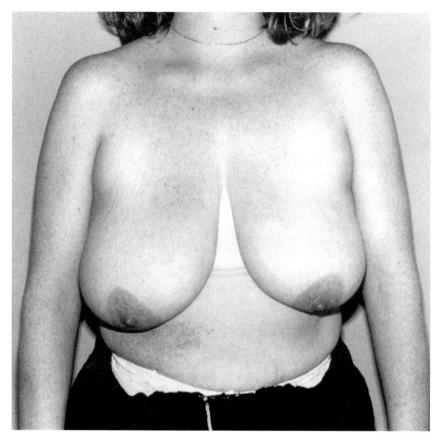

Patient Number:	*16*
Age:	37 years old
Incision Pattern:	Vertical

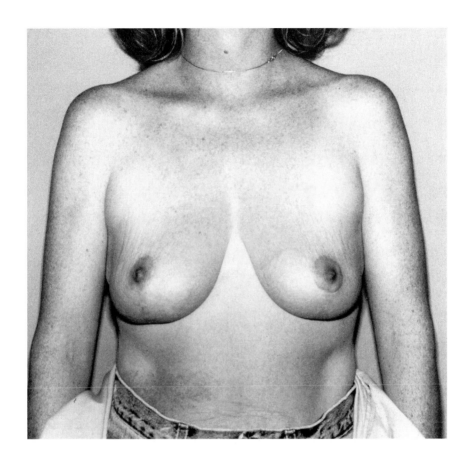

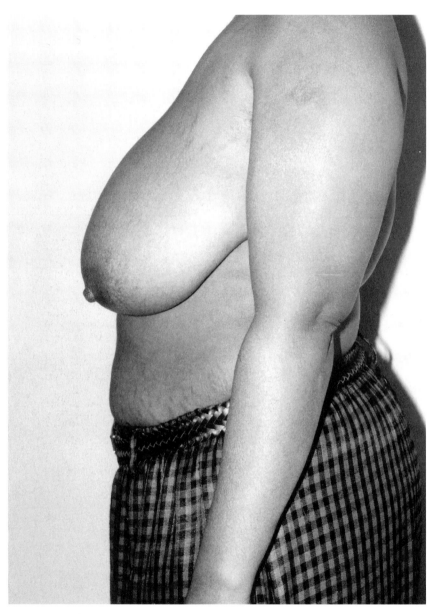

Patient Number: 17
Age: 32 years old
Incision: Anchor-shaped

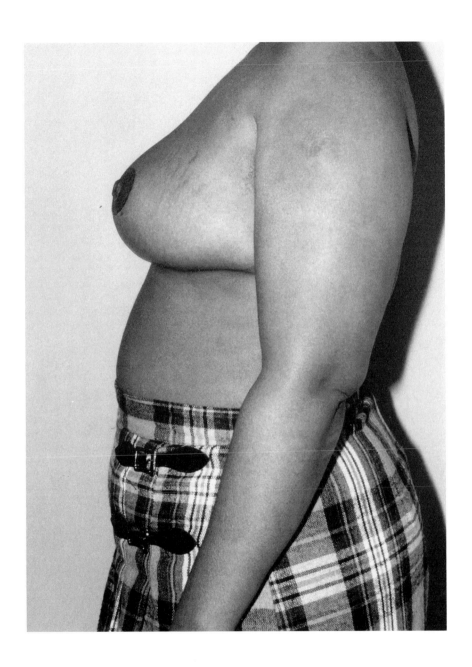

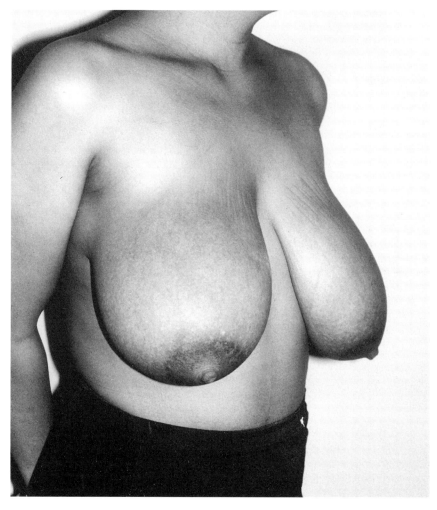

Patient Number:	*18*
Age:	29 years old
Incision Pattern:	Anchor-shaped

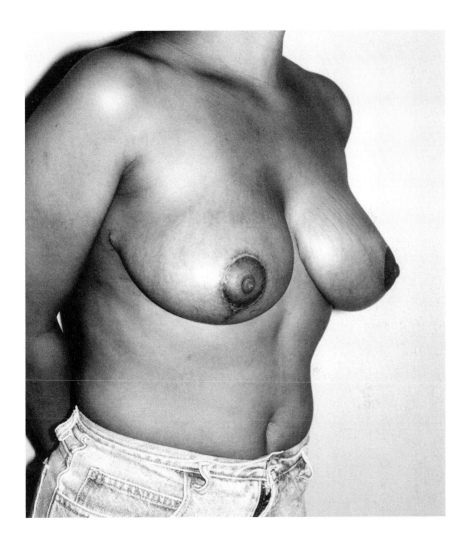

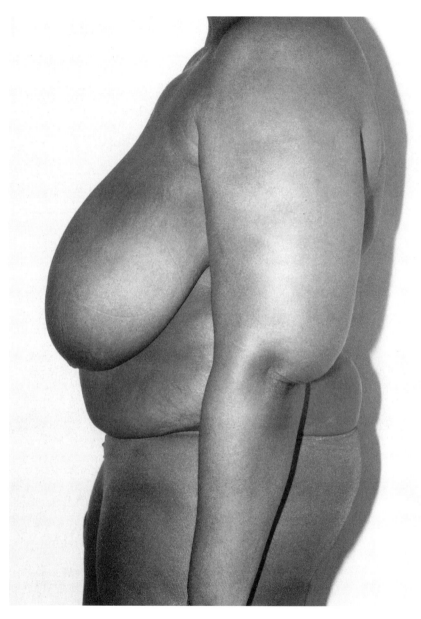

Patient Number: *19*
Age: 39 years old
Incision: Anchor-shaped

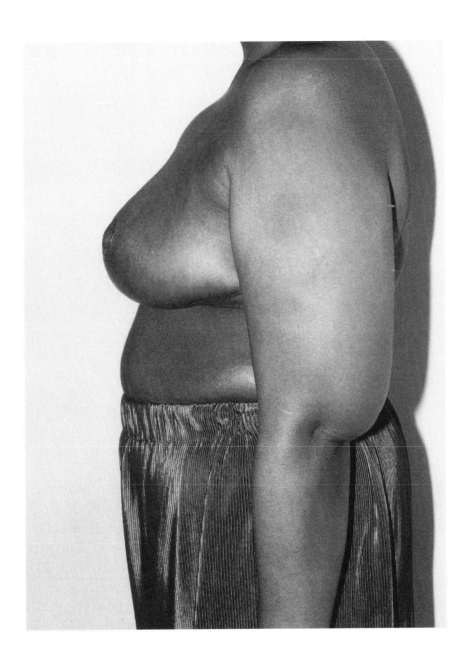

CHAPTER 38

Liposuction: The Face and Neck

Liposuction can be used to remove fat from any area of the face and neck, but the most common site is from under the chin (the "submental region"). It can be performed as an isolated procedure or in association with a facelift. When performed alone, it can often be done instead of a facelift. Its popularity has increased dramatically, as the recovery for this procedure is much less involved than for a facelift, and in many patients, the results are nearly as good. Typically, this is in younger patients (30s, 40s and early 50s) who have submental fat and some loose skin but relatively little extra skin elsewhere on the face. In addition, it is useful for some patients who would benefit from a facelift but who do not want one or who, for medical reasons, should not have one. In some patients, depending on the degree and location of excess skin, a facelift (including the liposuction) may be necessary in order to achieve an aesthetic result. In patients with tighter skin, liposuction alone can produce a dramatic improvement.

The incisions used (see Figures #4 and #5) are the submental and, occasionally, the postauricular (behind the ear). As with other procedures, the incisions are small (about 1/8 to 1/2 inch) and, with time, fade into unobtrusive scars. When liposuction is performed with or during a facelift, the standard facelift incisions (which are more extensive and are located in front of the ear, behind the ear, and into the hairline, in addition to the submental incision) are used. In addition to the removal of fat, adjunctive procedures that can be performed simultaneously include tightening of the muscles under the chin and insertion of a suture across the neckline that can further tighten and define the neck crease.

Other areas of the face that are commonly treated are the cheeks and the jowls. Intra-oral incisions (inside the mouth) may be used to treat the cheeks and jowls; the jowls can also be reached from the submental incision.

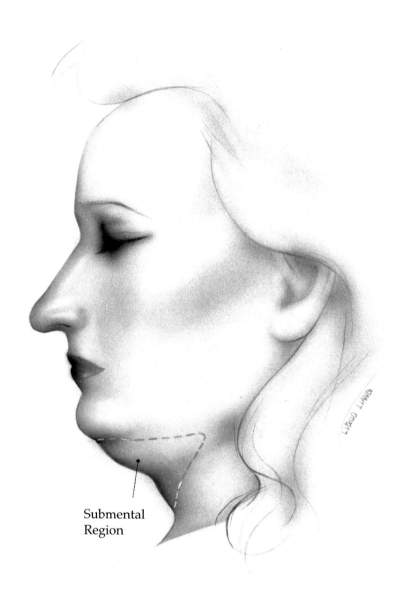

Submental
Region

Figure 4. Liposuction of Neck

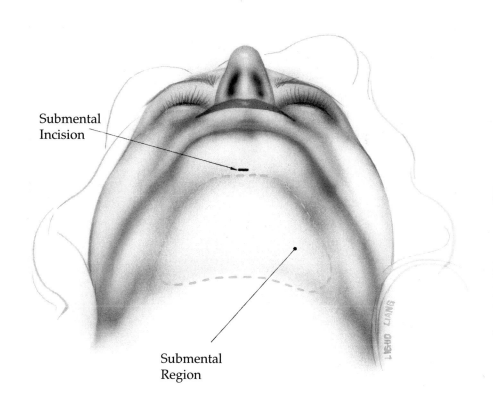

Submental
Incision

Submental
Region

Figure 5. Liposuction of Neck

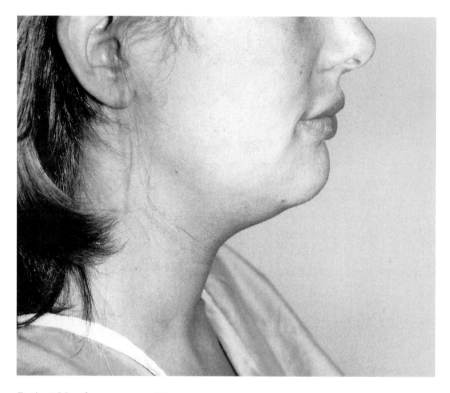

Patient Number :   *20*
Age: 25 years old
Incision: Submental

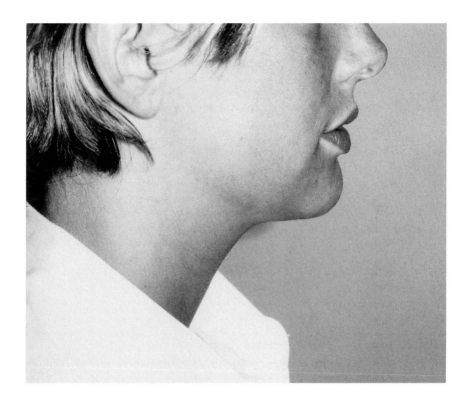

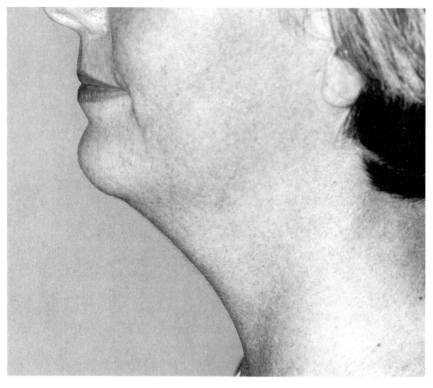

Patient Number: 21
Age: 34 years old
Incision: Submental

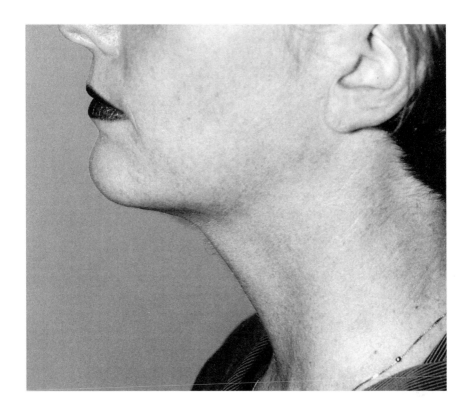

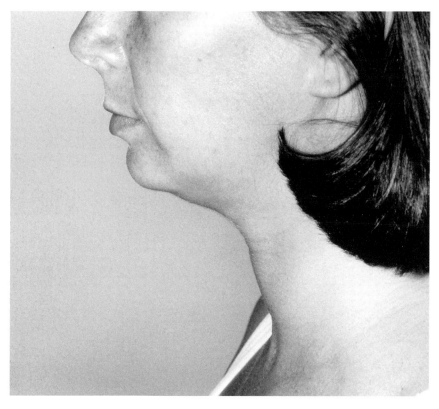

Patient Number: 22
Age: 31 years old
Incisions: Submental

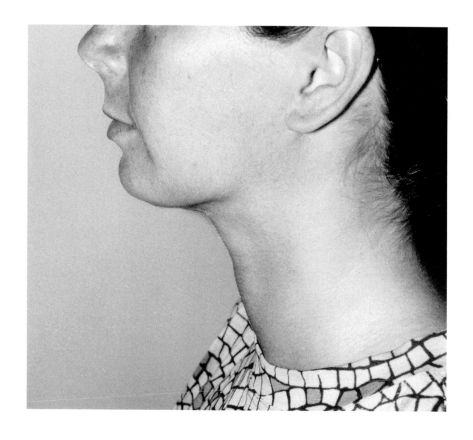

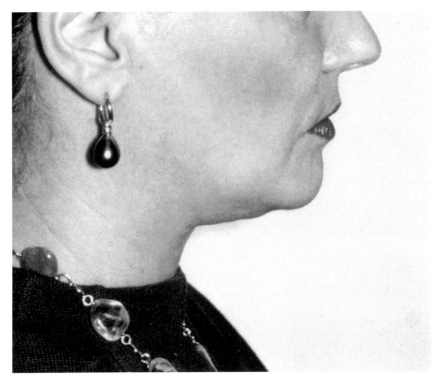

Patient Number :   23
Age: 49 years old
Incisions: Submental

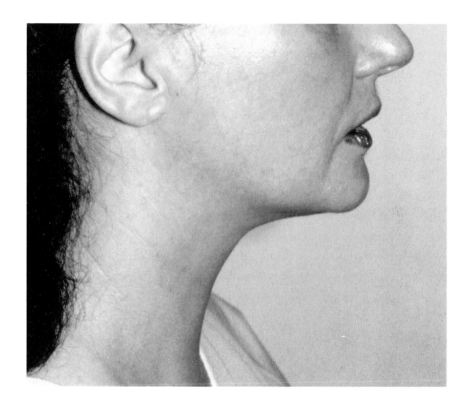

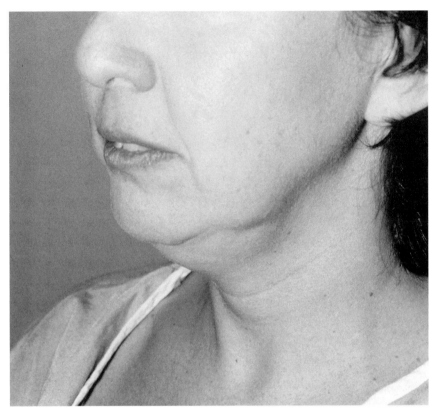

Patient Number: 24
Age: 43 years old
Incisions: Submental

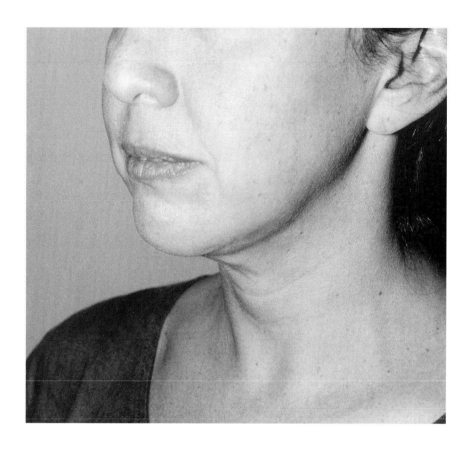

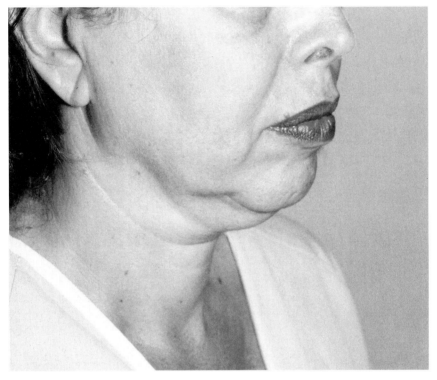

Patient Number: 25
Age: 45 years old
Incision: Submental

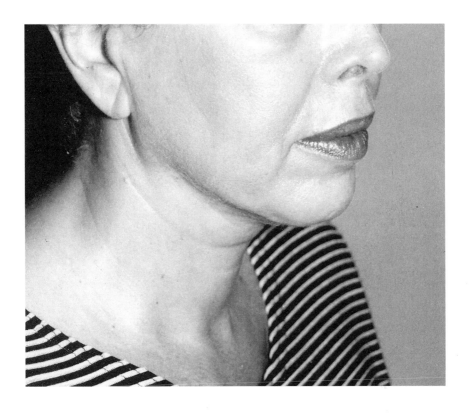

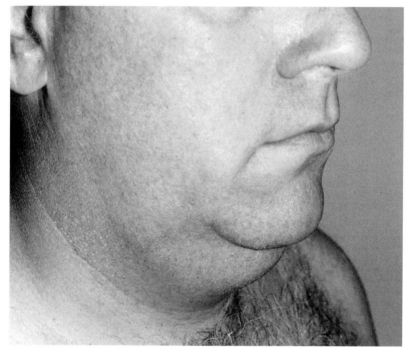

Patient Number:	26
Age:	48 years old
Incision:	Submental

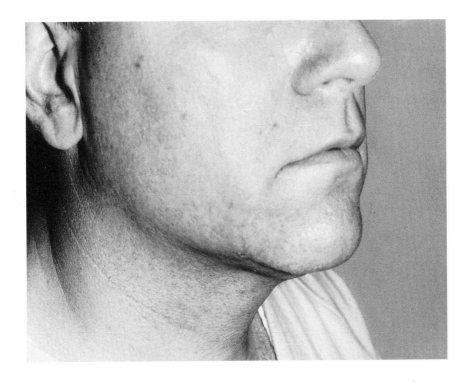

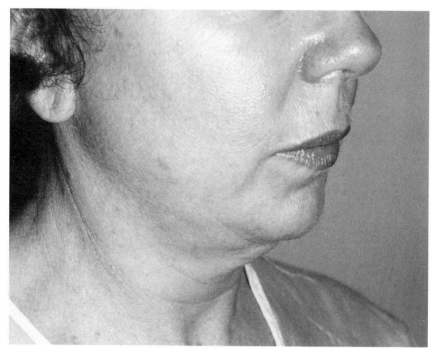

Patient Number: 27
Age: 52 years old
Incision: Submental

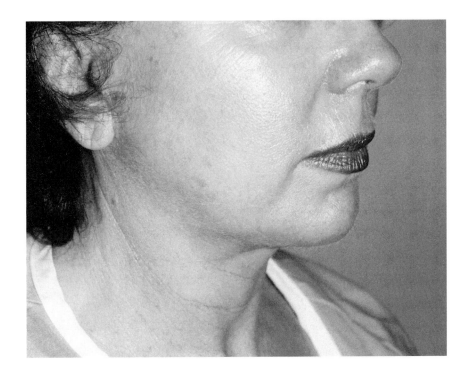

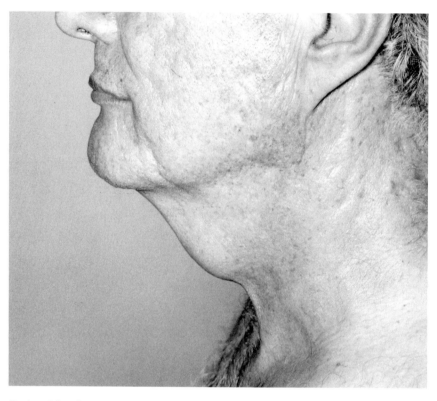

Patient Number:	*28*
Age:	63 years old
Incisions:	Submental

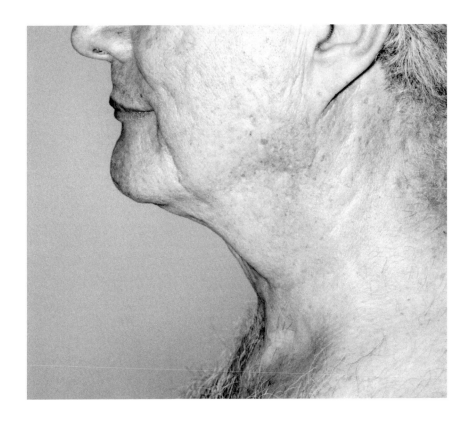

CHAPTER 39

Liposuction: Stomach, Hips, and Thighs

These areas represent the majority of the liposuction procedures performed and are shown in Figures #6 and #7. Few areas of the body are subject to such rapid, and sometimes drastic, changes as are the stomach and hips, particularly following one or more pregnancies. Some people are able to return to their pre-pregnancy shape, or nearly so; many are not. There are, as always, multiple explanations for this: heredity, weight gain during the pregnancy, number of pregnancies, etc. Regardless of the cause, one's body can undergo transformations that are not desirable. When the changes are characterized primarily by excess fat, liposuction can offer marked improvements. Many conditions, including those that previously were treated with tummy tucks, are now effectively treated with liposuction alone. The pictures speak for themselves, but even they do not always tell the whole story. Because of its three-dimensional and circumferential aspects, the total impact of liposuction is often greater than the photos alone would suggest.

For liposuction of the stomach and the extended stomach (see diagram), one or two incisions hidden within the belly button (umbilical incision) and within the pubic hair (pubic) are used. In some cases, extra incisions are required; whenever possible existing scars (e.g., appendectomy, Caesarean section) are used.

In general, both the thighs (outer and inner) and the hips can be recontoured using one incision on each side. The scar that results from this incision, which measures up to about 1/2 inch, is hidden within the crease under the buttock (infragluteal). It is located about 1/4 to 1/3 of the way from the inner to the outer thigh. Many surgeons use several incisions, placed circumferentially around a given region and in potentially visible locations, attempting to remove fat from more than one angle. As previously discussed, this is normally not necessary, and there are reasons to limit the number of incisions used. With the exception of Patients #49 and #50, the results shown here were achieved using a *single* incision for the thighs and hips, thereby avoiding scars in visible areas.

These regions (stomach, hips, and thighs) are often treated together in order to achieve the maximum improvement in contour. This should be individualized, and isolated deformities (particularly of the stomach or outer thighs) are effectively treated with more limited procedures. As previously noted, it may be advantageous to recontour additional regions, even if there is one in particular that was the "target." With respect to the thighs, the outer portions tend to be the most amenable to correction by liposuction. This is followed by the inner thighs and, to a lesser degree, the front and back of the thighs, and the buttocks. These differences in ease of correction are due primarily to differences in anatomy, i.e., the qualities of the skin, fat, and subcutaneous tissue in each of the areas. As with the anterior knees and calves (see below), the relatively superficial nature of the fat of the anterior thigh means that liposuction in this region has an increased risk of visible postoperative contour irregularities.

An increasingly popular area for recontouring is the back, both upper and lower. Excess fat in this region may be noticeable depending on the type of clothing (specifically the bra) or bathing suit top worn. The elastic in these garments compresses the skin and pushes the fat into increased prominence; this is often visible through outer clothing. These areas respond well to liposuction, although the relatively large amount of dense, fibrous subcutaneous tissue in this region limits, somewhat, the results that can be achieved.

Furthermore, one or more small incisions in potentially visible sites may be required on each side.

For each of the following cases, the areas treated are listed; as is commonly seen, some areas show more dramatic improvement than others, even within the same patient. In general, the overall effect is more profound when more areas are treated.

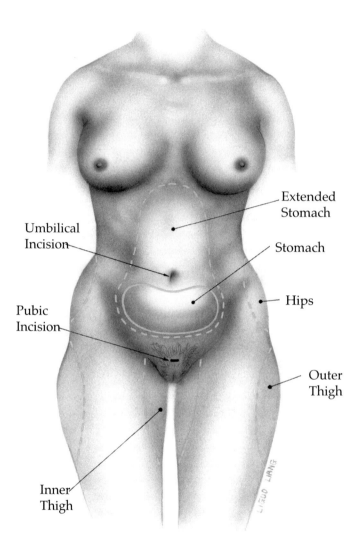

Extended
Stomach

Umbilical
Incision

Stomach

Pubic
Incision

Hips

Outer
Thigh

Inner
Thigh

Figure 6.   Liposuction of Stomach

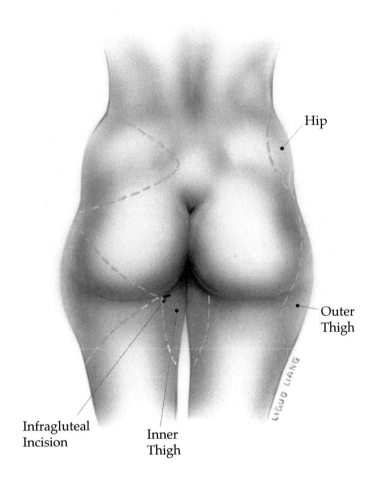

Hip

Outer
Thigh

Infragluteal
Incision

Inner
Thigh

Figure 7. Liposuction of Hips and Thighs

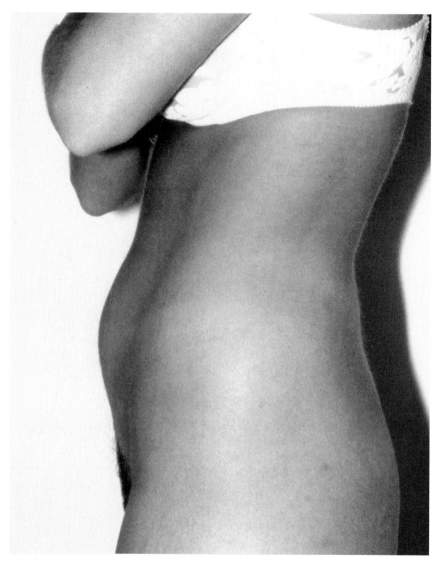

Patient Number:	*29*
Age:	26 years old
Areas:	Stomach, Hips, Thighs
Incisions:	Umbilical, Infragluteal

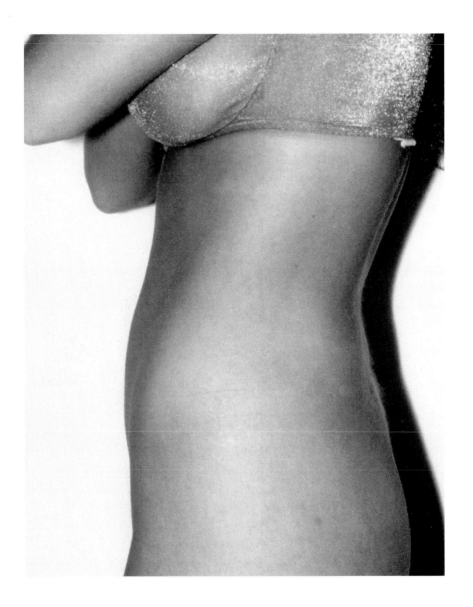

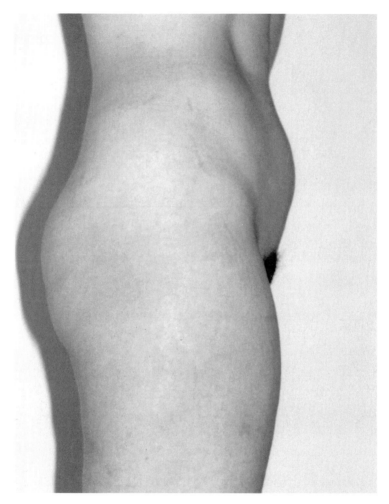

Patient Number:	*30*
Age:	30 years old
Areas:	Stomach, Hips, Thighs
Incisions:	Umbilical, Infragluteal

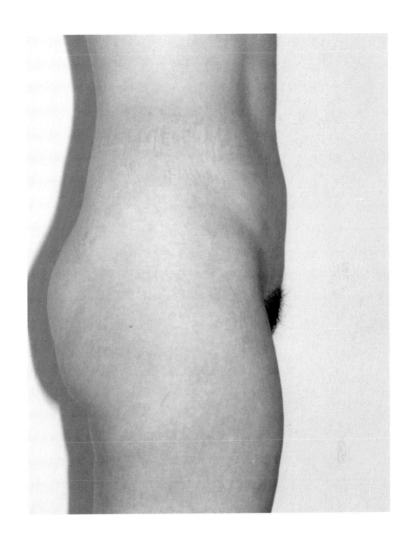

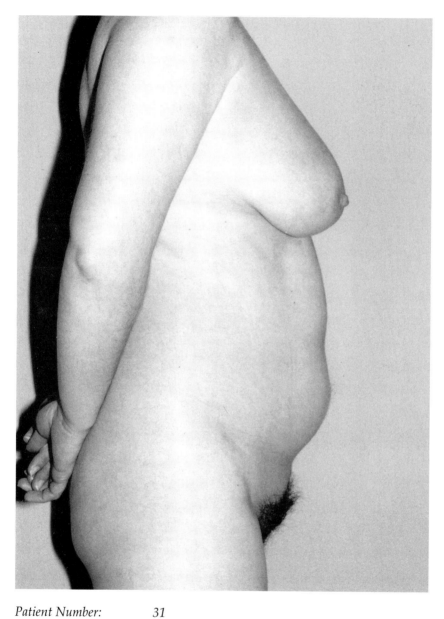

Patient Number:	31
Age:	37 years old
Areas:	Stomach, Hips, Thighs
Incisions:	Umbilical, Pubic

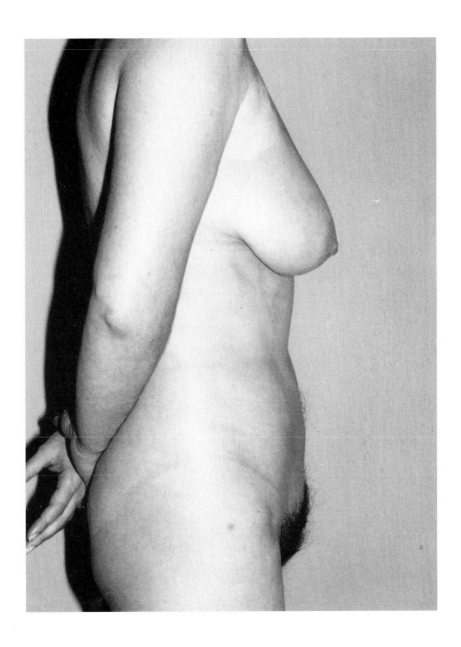

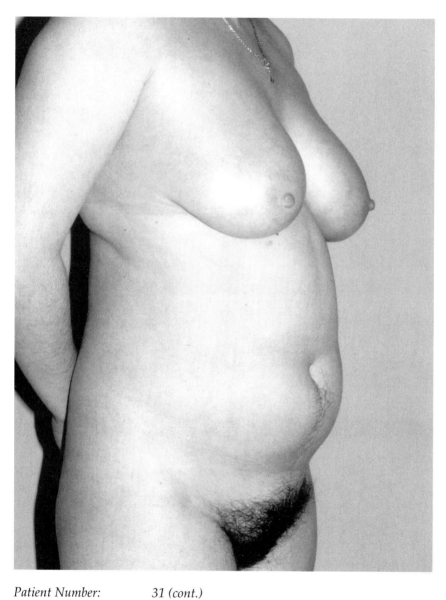

Patient Number:	31 (cont.)
Age:	37 years old
Area:	Stomach
Incision:	Umbilical, Pubic

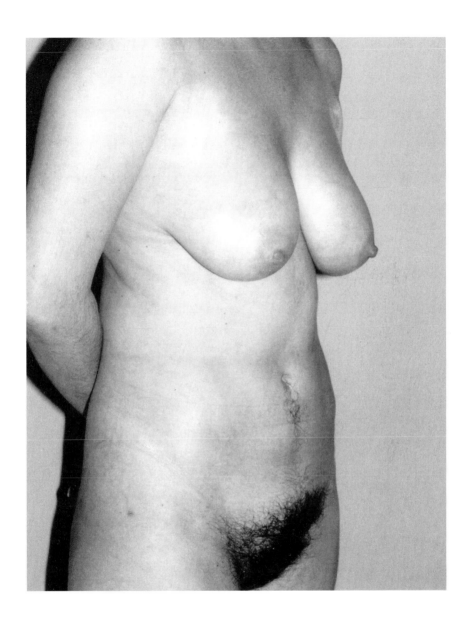

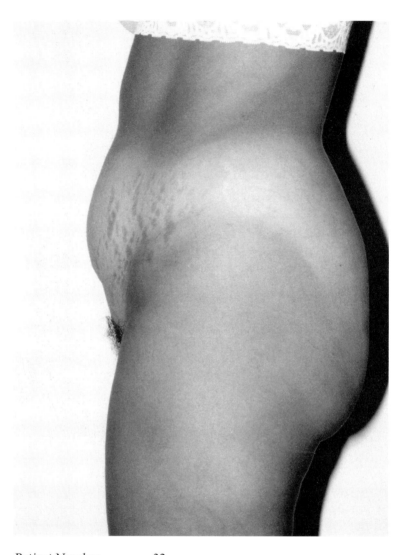

Patient Number: 32
Age: 29 years old
Areas: Stomach, Hips, Thighs
Incisions: Umbilical, Pubic, Infragluteal

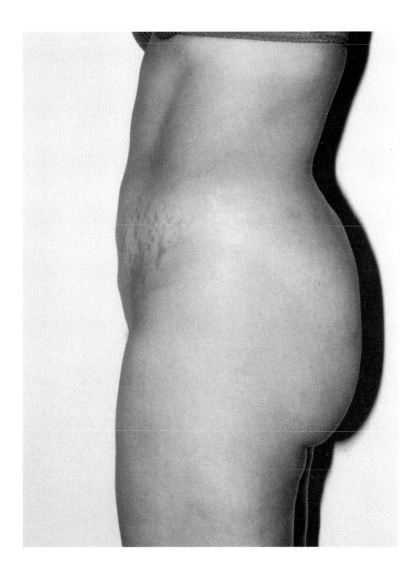

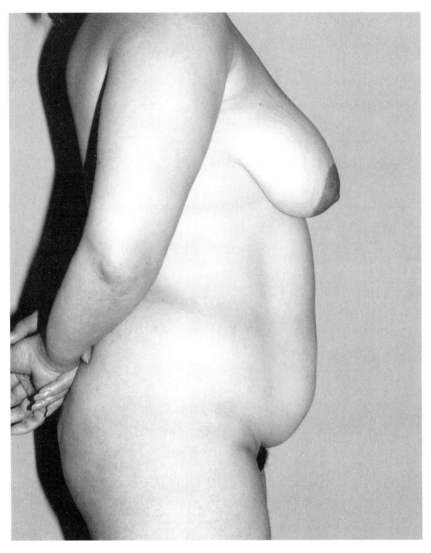

Patient Number:	33
Age:	37 years old
Areas:	Stomach, Hips, Thighs
Incisions:	Umbilical, Infragluteal

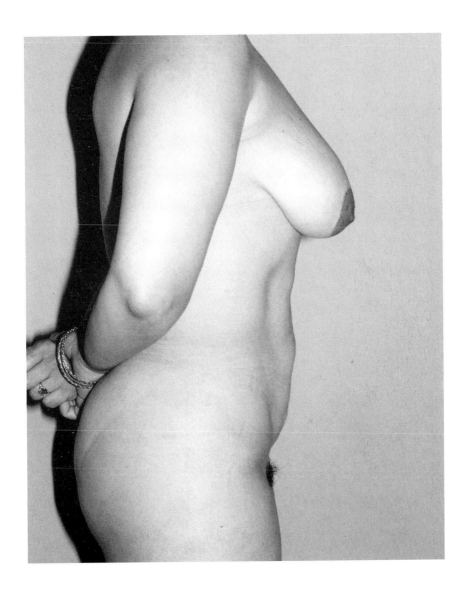

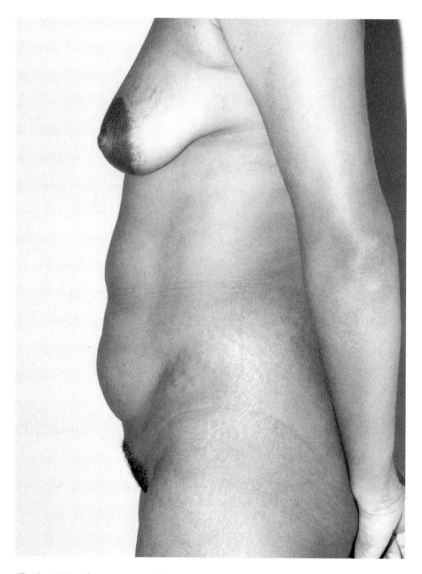

Patient Number:	*34*
Age:	29 years old
Areas:	Stomach, Hips, Thighs
Incisions:	Umbilical, Infragluteal

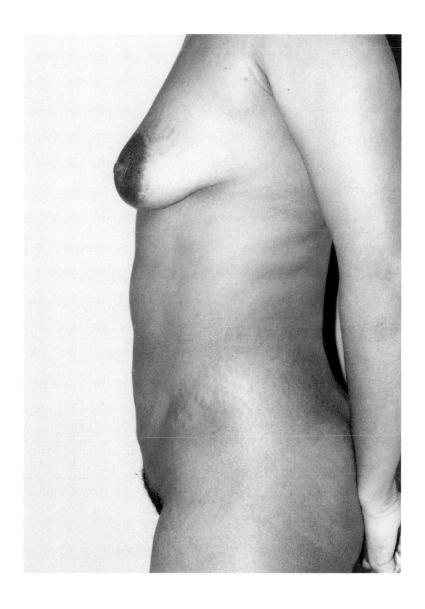

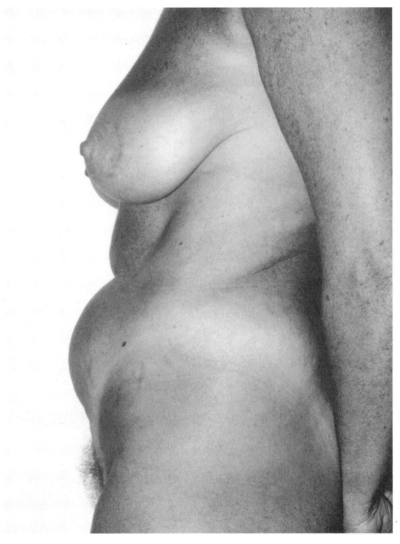

Patient Number:	*35*
Age:	48 years old
Areas:	Stomach, Hips, Thighs
Incisions:	Umbilical, Infragluteal

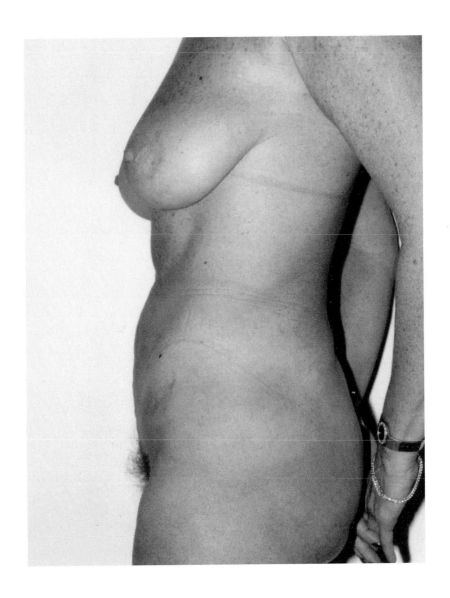

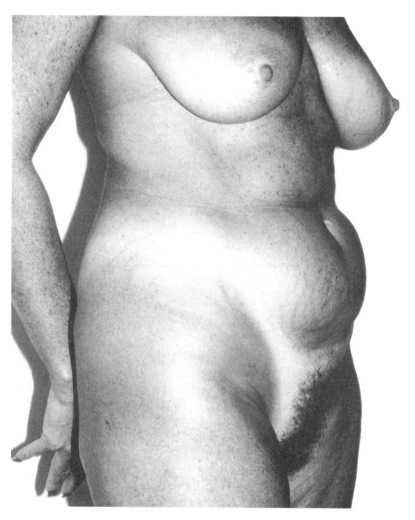

Patient Number:	*35 (cont.)*
Age:	48 years old
Areas:	Stomach, Hips, Thighs
Incisions:	Umbilical, Infragluteal

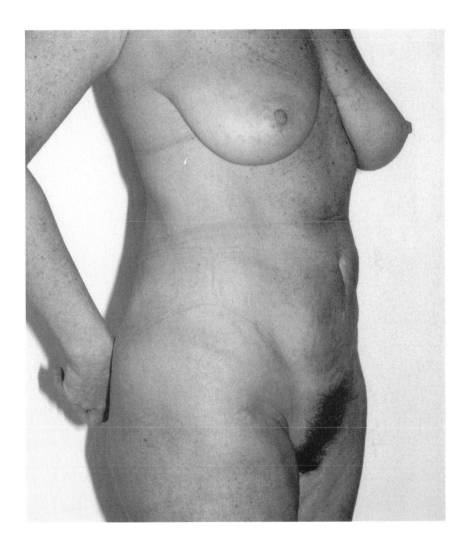

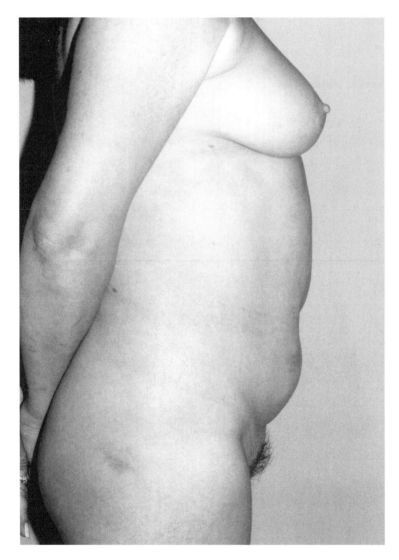

Patient Number: 36
Age: 51 years old
Areas: Stomach
Incisions: Umbilical, Pubic

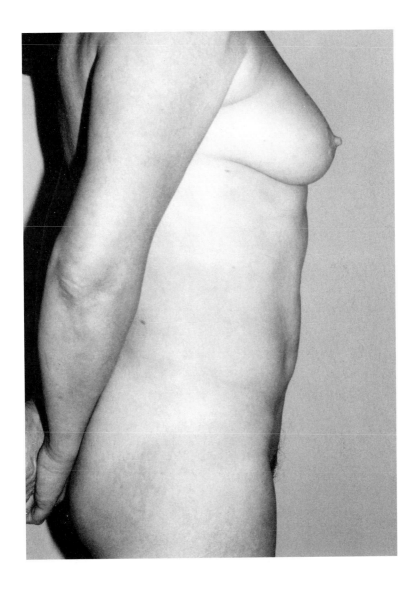

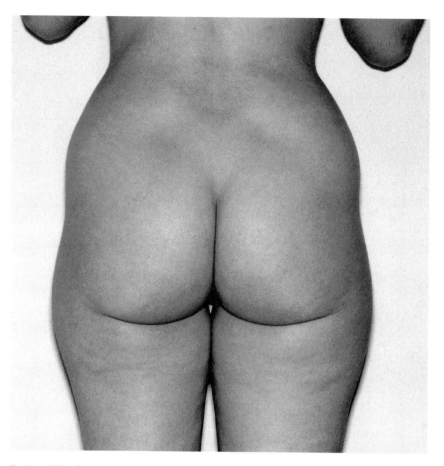

Patient Number:	37
Age:	22 years old
Areas:	Stomach, Hips, Thighs
Incisions:	Umbilical, Infragluteal

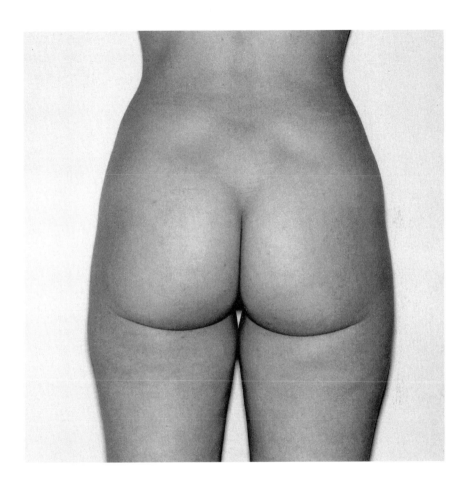

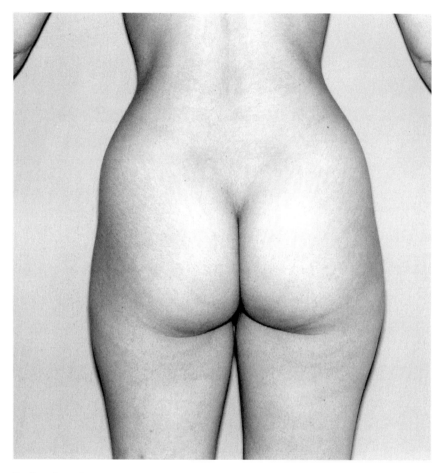

Patient Number:	*38*
Age:	25 years old
Areas:	Stomach, Hips, Thighs
Incision:	Umbilical, Infragluteal

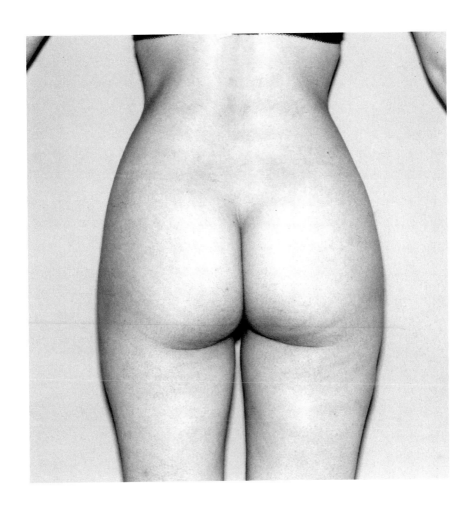

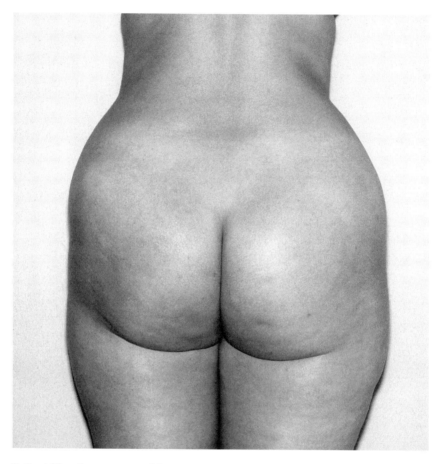

Patient Number: 39
Age: 27 years old
Areas: Stomach, Hips, Thighs
Incision: Umbilical, Infragluteal

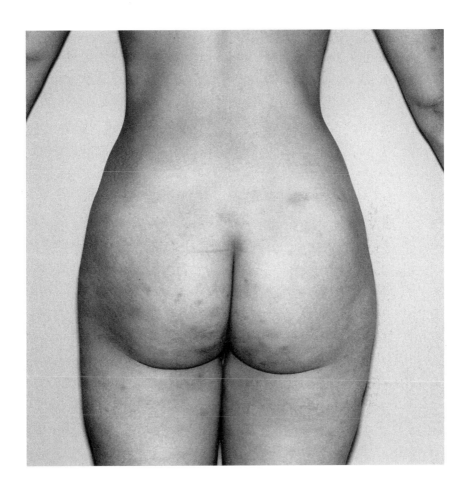

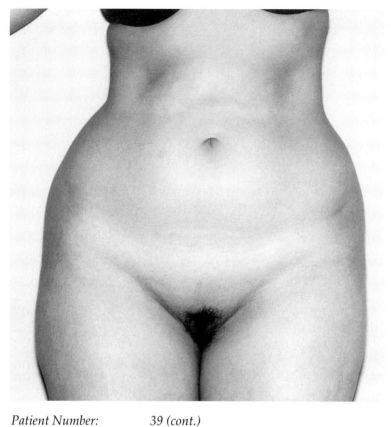

Patient Number: 39 (cont.)
Age: 27 years old
Areas: Stomach, Hips, Thighs
Incision: Umbilical, Infragluteal

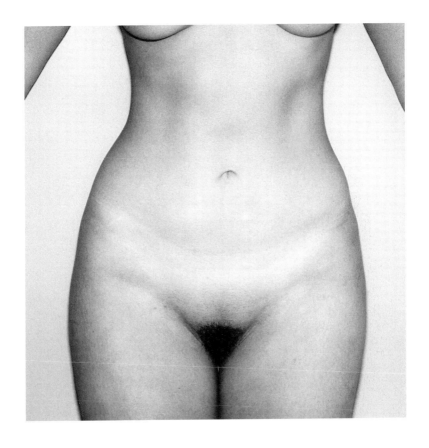

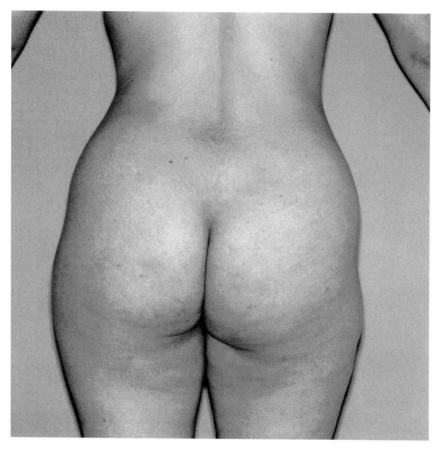

Patient Number:	*40*
Age:	35 years old
Areas:	Stomach, Hips, Thighs
Incisions:	Umbilical, Infragluteal

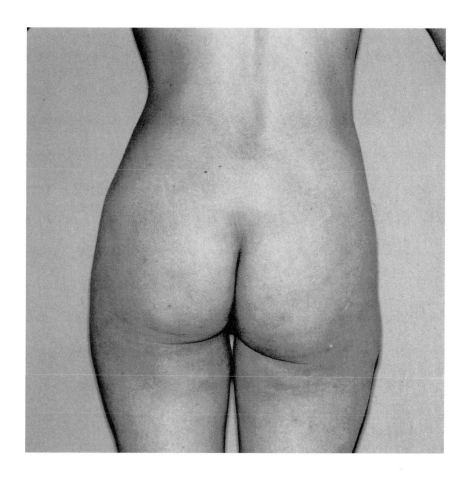

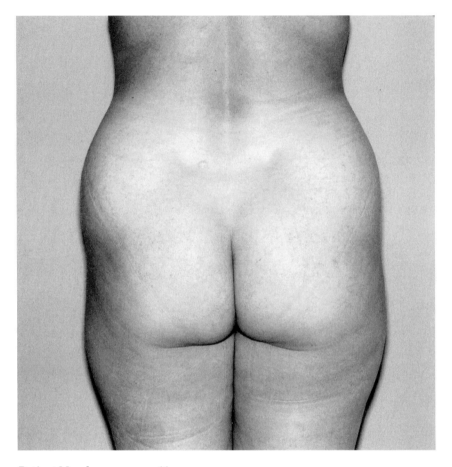

Patient Number:	*41*
Age:	34 years old
Areas:	Stomach, Hips, Thighs
Incisions:	Umbilical, Infragluteal

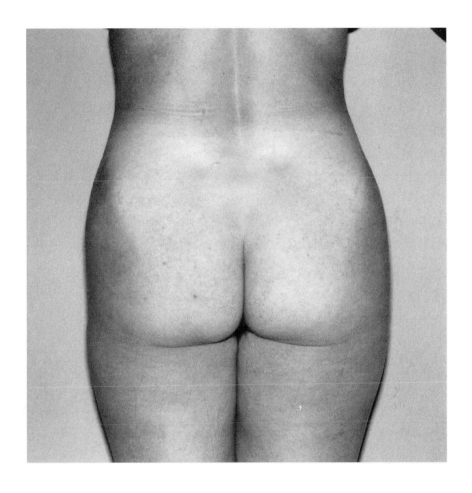

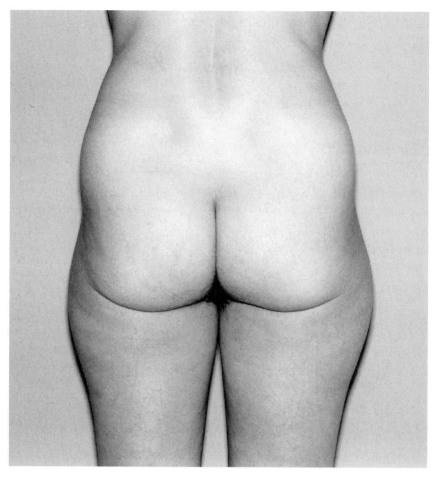

Patient Number: 42
Age: 38 years old
Areas: Hips, Thighs
Incisions: Infragluteal

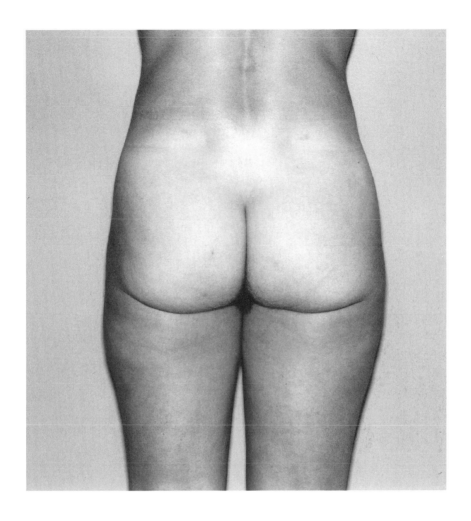

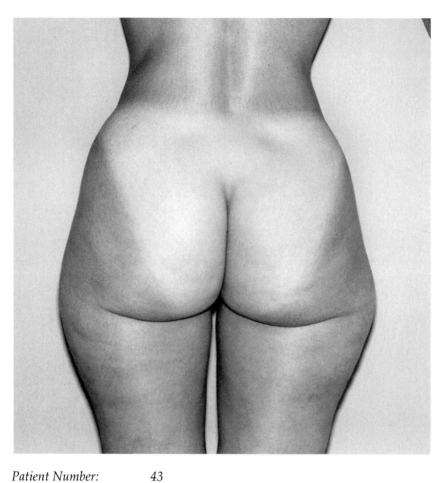

Patient Number: 43
Age: 35 years old
Areas: Hips, Thighs
Incision: Infragluteal

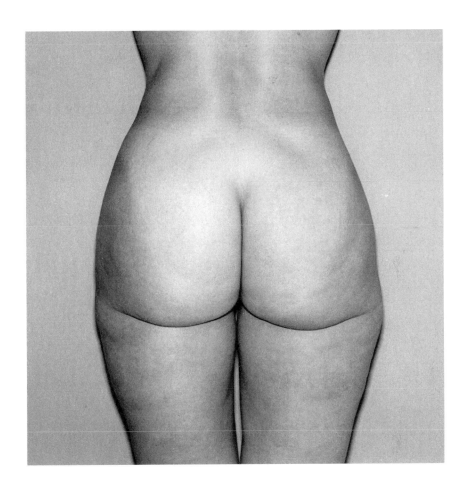

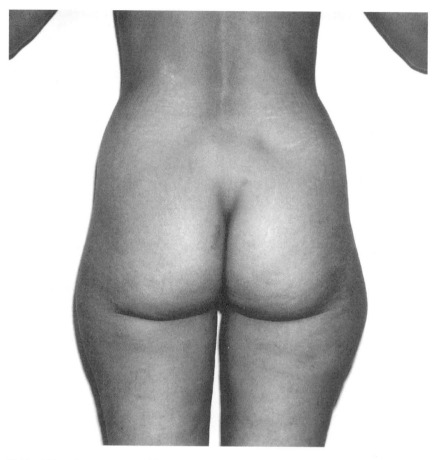

Patient Number:	*44*
Age:	39 years old
Areas:	Stomach, Hips, Thighs
Incisions:	Umbilical, Infragluteal

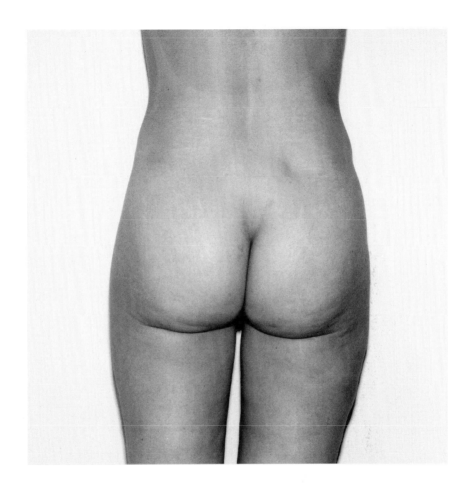

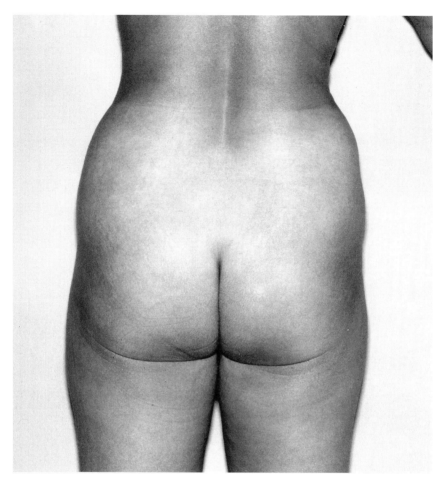

Patient Number:	45
Age:	39 years old
Areas:	Stomach, Hips, Thighs
Incisions:	Umbilical, Infragluteal

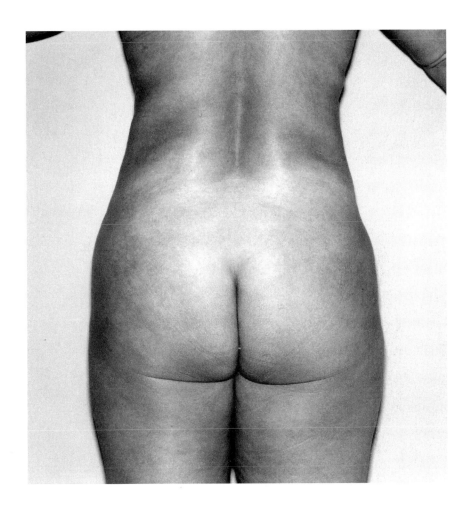

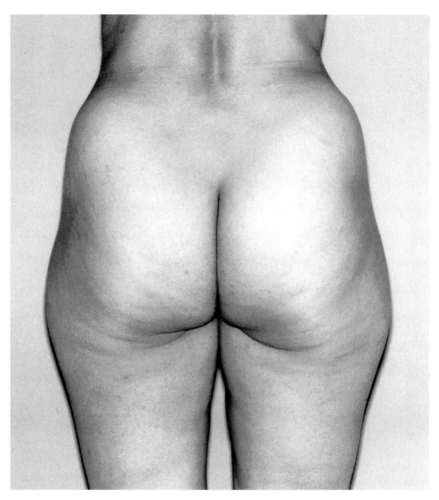

Patient Number: 46
Age: 47 years old
Areas: Stomach, Hips, Thighs
Incisions: Umbilical, Infragluteal

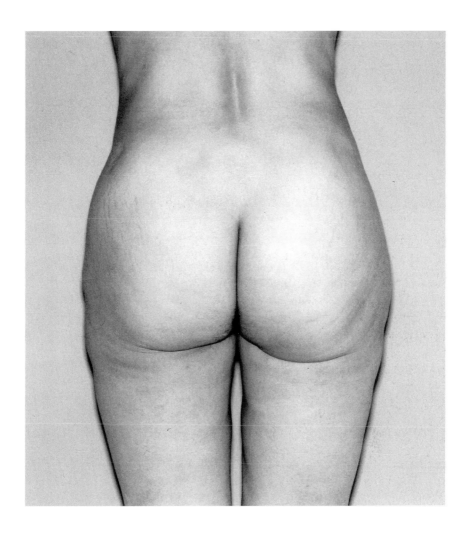

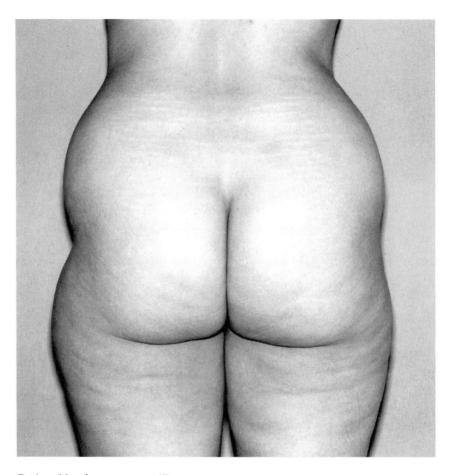

Patient Number:	*47*
Age:	34 years old
Areas:	Hips, Thighs
Incisions:	Infragluteal (also had Tummy Tuck)

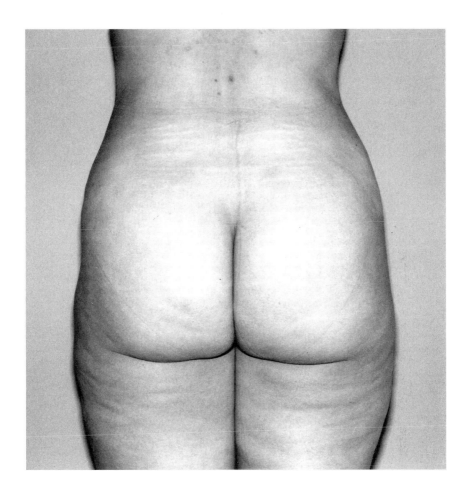

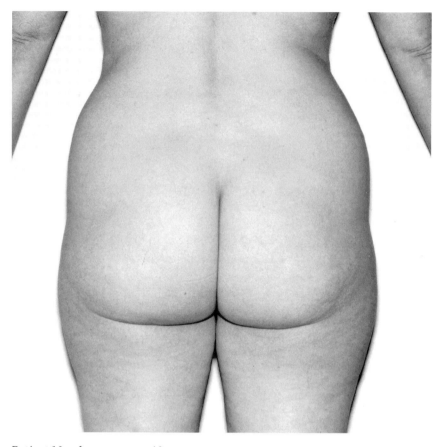

Patient Number: 48
Age: 48 years old
Areas: Stomach, Hips, Thighs
Incisions: Umbilical, Infragluteal

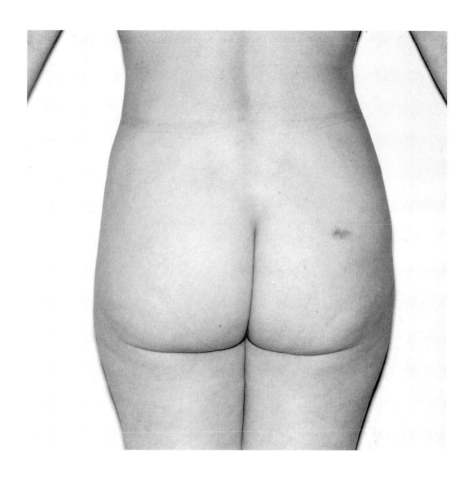

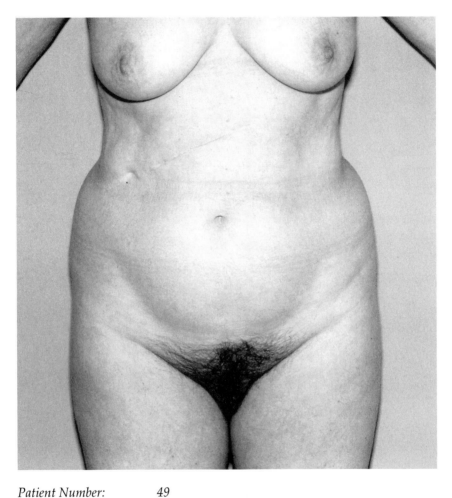

Patient Number:	*49*
Age:	53 years old
Areas:	Stomach, Hips, Thighs
Incisions:	Umbilical, Infragluteal, Hip

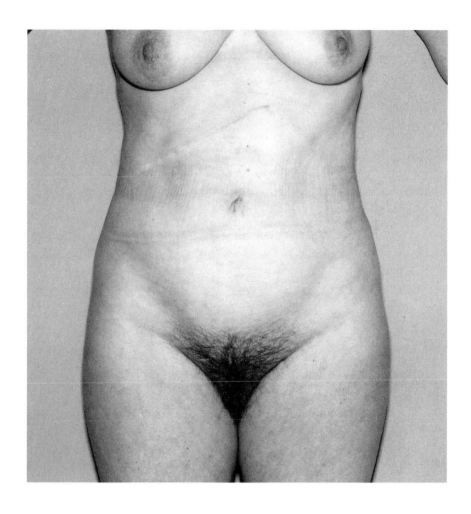

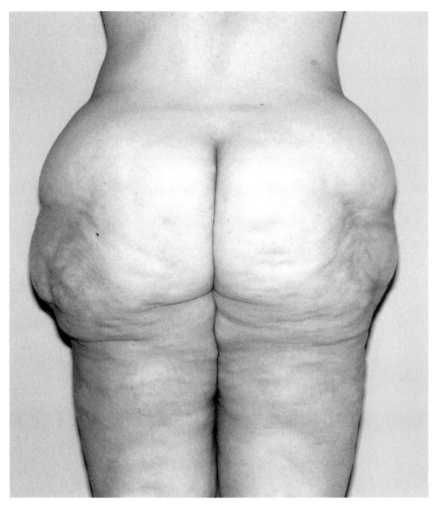

Patient Number:	*50*
Age:	44 years old
Areas:	Stomach, Hips, Thighs
Incisions:	Umbilical, Infragluteal, Hip

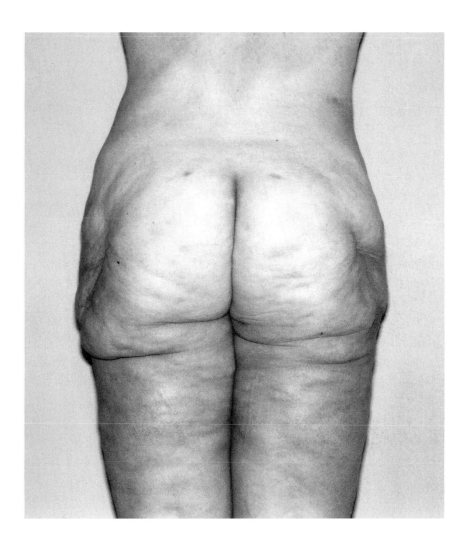

CHAPTER 40

Liposuction: Knees, Calves, and Ankles

If the "bumps" on the inner knees are made up largely of fat, they may be treated with liposuction. A single incision in the natural crease behind each knee (popliteal) is used to reshape the contour (see Figure #8). If the bumps are due largely to bony protrusions, liposuction will not be successful; if there is a large amount of extra skin, liposuction may not be advisable. The region of the front of the knees is another area of popular concern. This can be more difficult to treat, however, as the skin tends to be relatively loose. This increases the likelihood of postoperative skin irregularities. Again, each patient is examined, and based on the anatomy and the patient's goals, an individual treatment plan is formulated.

The calves and ankles can also be treated with liposuction, since these regions of the legs are exposed with nearly all dress lengths. Normally, 2 to 4 small incisions are required on each side. Although the procedure is effective, the fat in this portion of the anatomy is relatively superficial and tends to be somewhat fibrous. The visibility of the region makes the risk of irregularities somewhat more of a concern than with most other regions. Finally, due presumably to the effects of gravity, it usually takes a relatively long time for swelling to subside in these regions. Despite this, the benefits of the correction of these areas in good candidates far outweighs the somewhat prolonged and uncomfortable recovery.

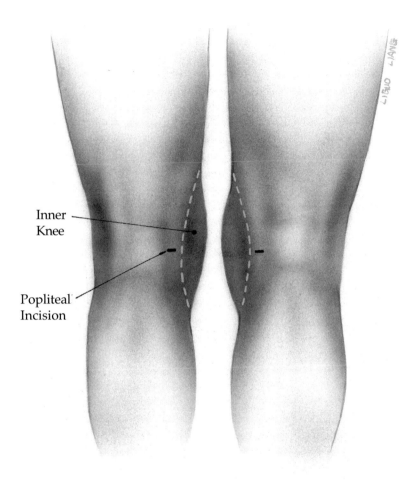

Inner Knee

Popliteal Incision

Figure 8. Liposuction of Knees

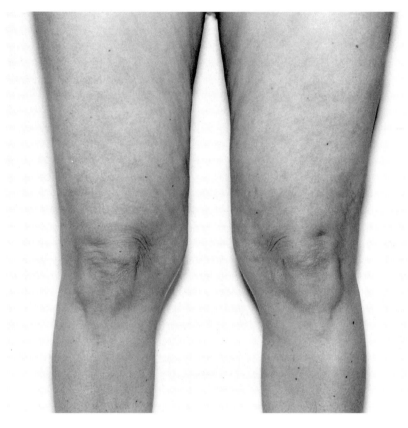

Patient Number:	51
Age:	44 years old
Areas:	Inner Knees
Incisions:	Knee

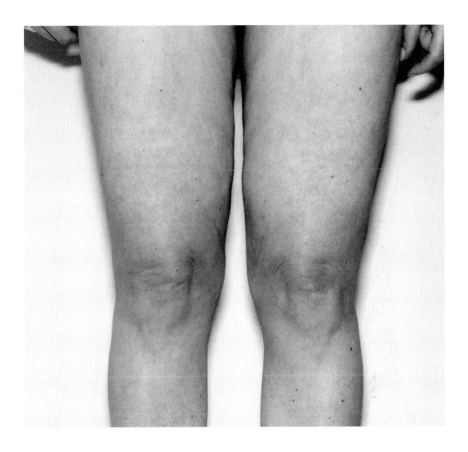

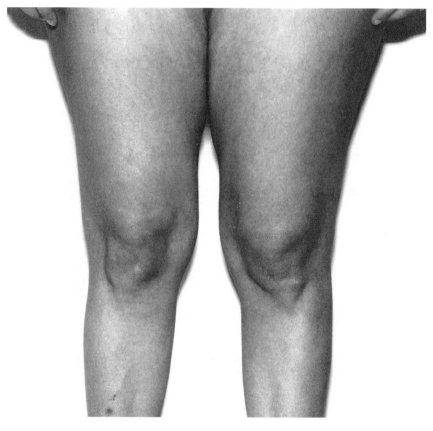

Patient Number:	*52*
Age:	36 years old
Areas:	Thighs, Inner Knees
Incisions:	Infragluteal, Knee

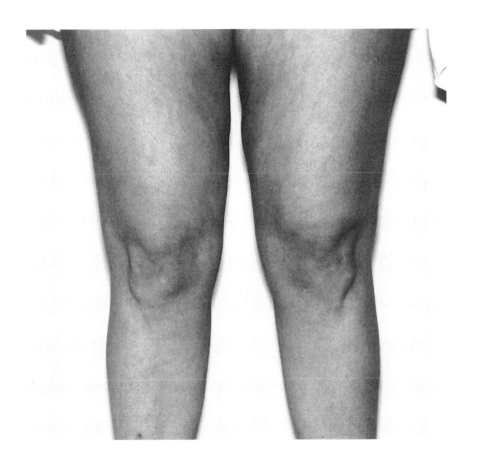

CHAPTER 41

Liposuction: Men — Chest, Stomach, and Love Handles

The treatment of the stomach in men is similar to that in women, although the accumulations of fat may be in slightly different areas (love handles), and therefore, different or additional incisions may be required (see Figure #9). Furthermore, the skin and subcutaneous tissue tend to be particularly thick and dense (when compared with that of a woman). Because of this difference in skin thickness, an area of "excess" may not be quite as thin postoperatively as would a similar area on a woman. Nevertheless, liposuction can produce dramatic contour changes in the areas being treated. Fat that is intra-abdominal (which is fairly common in men and can be determined during a physical examination) is not accessible to liposuction. Even then, there may be enough subcutaneous fat so that, once removed, improvement can be expected. As always, the key factors are the amount and distribution of the fat.

For male breasts (gynecomastia), the only incisions usually required are hidden within the axilla (i.e., under the arm). Occasionally, an additional incision located at the lower part of the areola (the dark area around the nipple) is necessary. Typically, these scars fade within several months and may be hidden within chest hair. Male breasts are composed of varying amounts of both fat and breast tissue. An increased percentage of fat versus breast tissue correspondingly increases the likelihood of success using liposuction alone.

In addition, the amount of excess skin must be considered. When there is not too much loose skin, the breasts can normally be reshaped using liposuction alone. If there is significant laxity (looseness) of the skin, such as after a major weight loss (100 pounds or more), or when the breasts are composed of particularly dense tissue, liposuction alone may not provide adequate treatment. In these cases, liposuction is combined with a skin resection and/or a wider incision to remove the breast tissue. The majority of gynecomastia cases, however, can be corrected with liposuction alone.

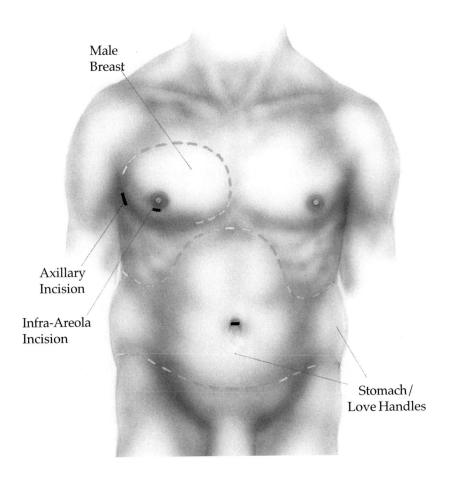

Male
Breast

Axillary
Incision

Infra-Areola
Incision

Stomach/
Love Handles

Figure 9.   Liposuction, Men (Chest, Stomach and Love Handles)

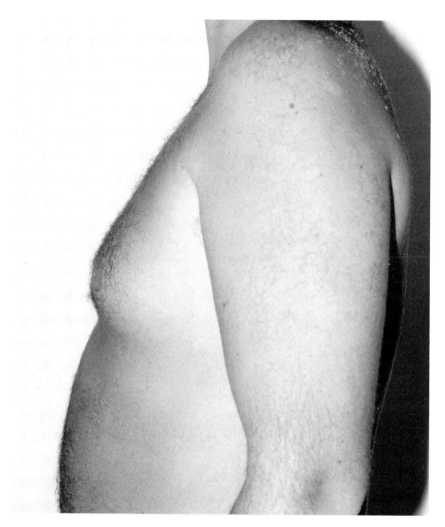

Patient Number:	*53*
Age:	31 years old
Areas:	Chest, Stomach, Lovehandles
Incisions:	Axillary, Umbilical, Groin

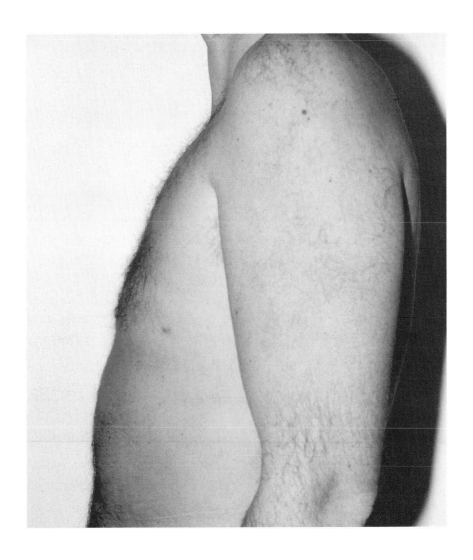

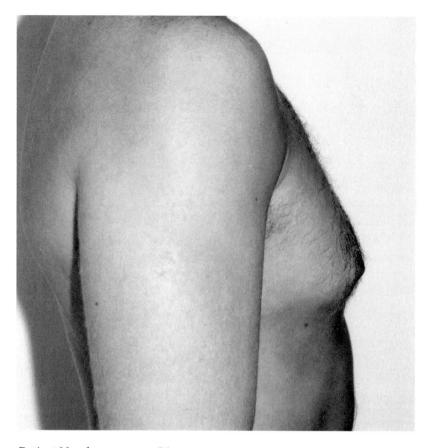

Patient Number:	*54*
Age:	26 years old
Areas:	Chest
Incisions:	Axillary

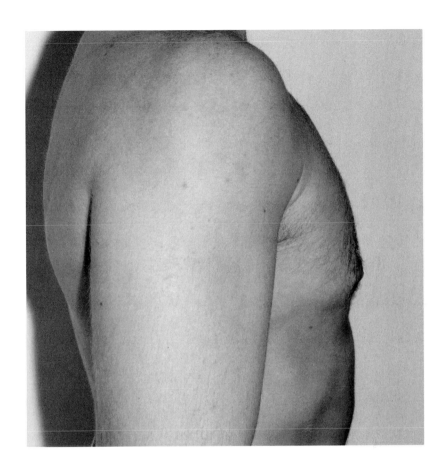

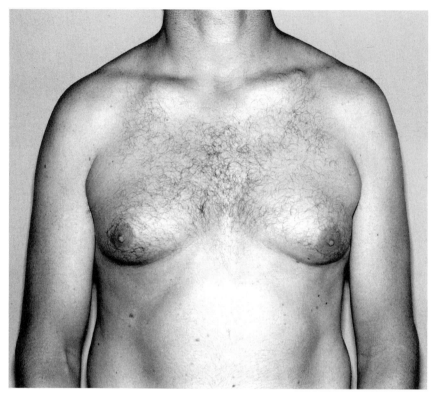

Patient Number:	*55*
Age:	43 years old
Areas:	Chest
Incisions:	Axillary

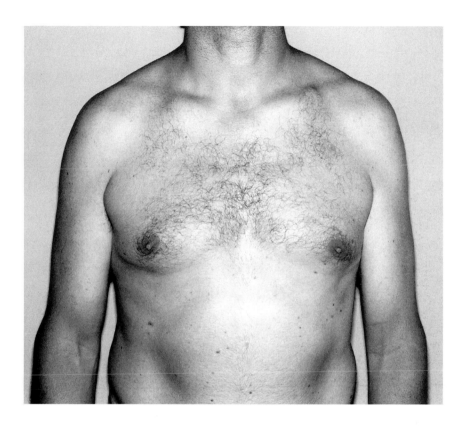

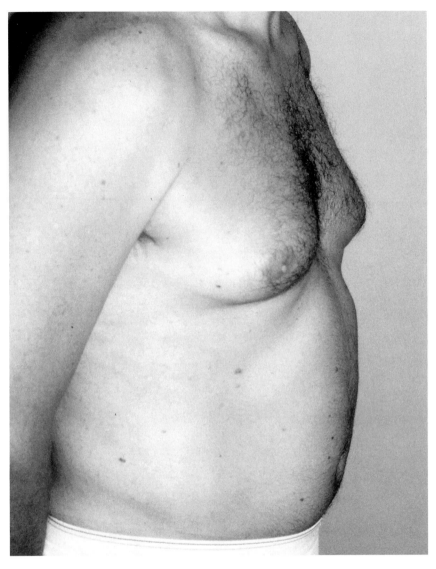

Patient Number: 55 (cont.)
Age: 43 years old
Areas: Chest
Incisions: Axillary

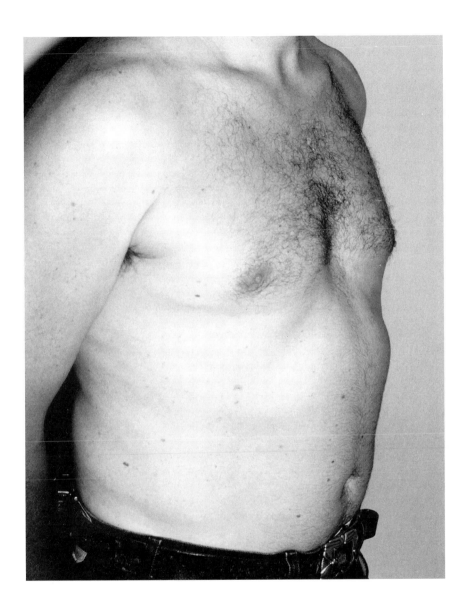

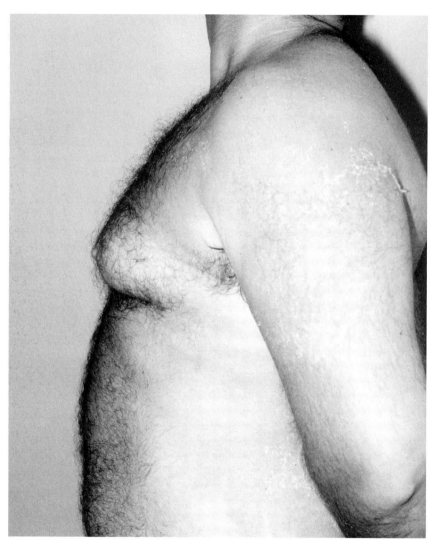

Patient Number: 56
Age: 38 years old
Areas: Chest
Incisions: Axillary

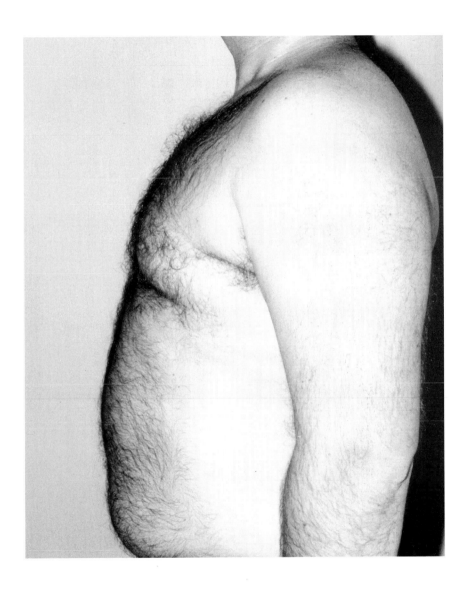

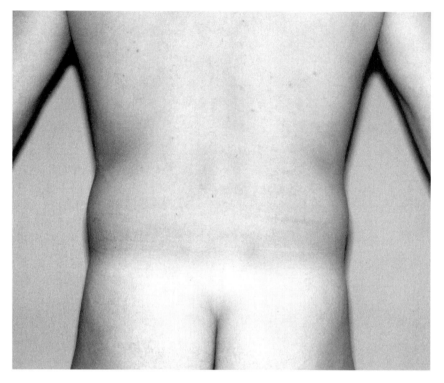

Patient Number:	*57*
Age:	29 years old
Areas:	Stomach, Lovehandles
Incisions:	Umbilical, Groin

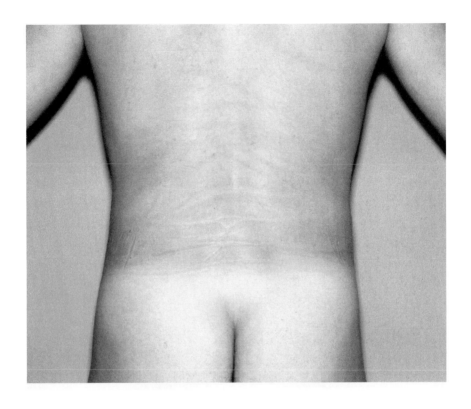

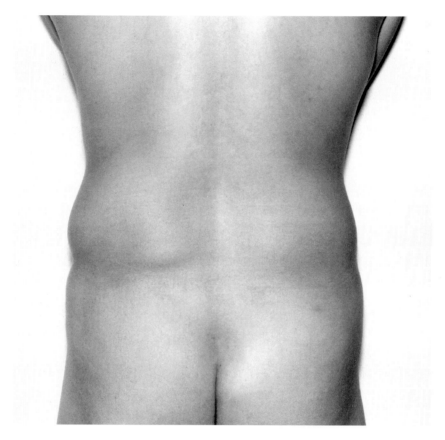

Patient Number:	*58*
Age:	43 years old
Areas:	Stomach, Lovehandles
Incisions:	Umbilical, Groin

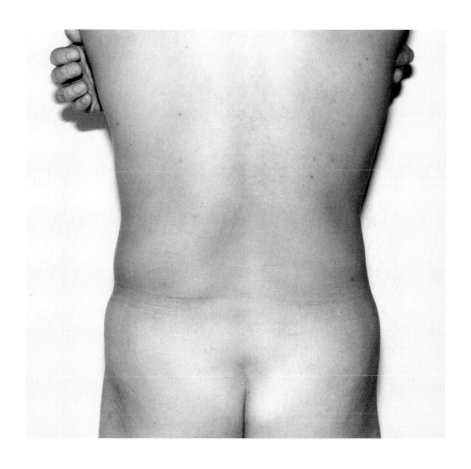

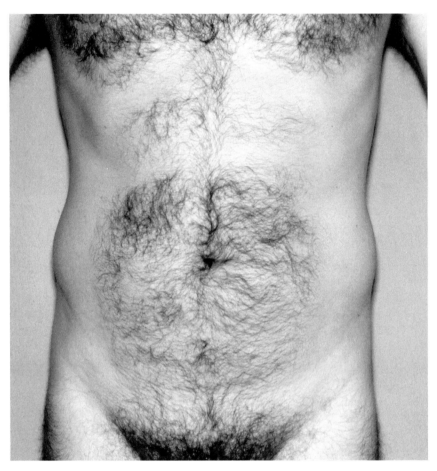

Patient Number:	*59*
Age:	38 years old
Areas:	Stomach, Lovehandles
Incisions:	Umbilical, Groin

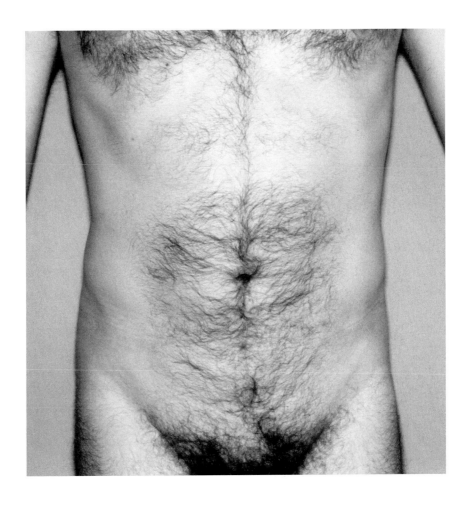

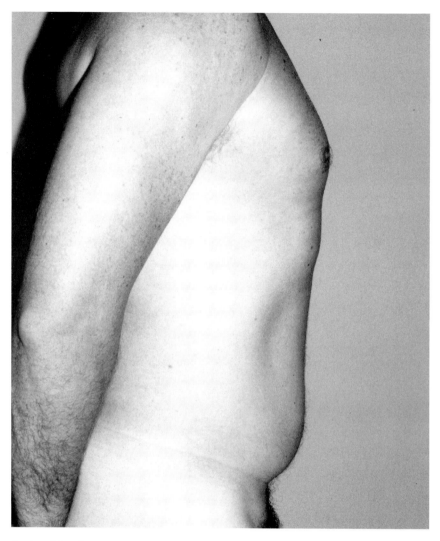

Patient Number: 60
Age: 38 years old
Areas: Stomach, Lovehandles
Incisions: Umbilical, Groin

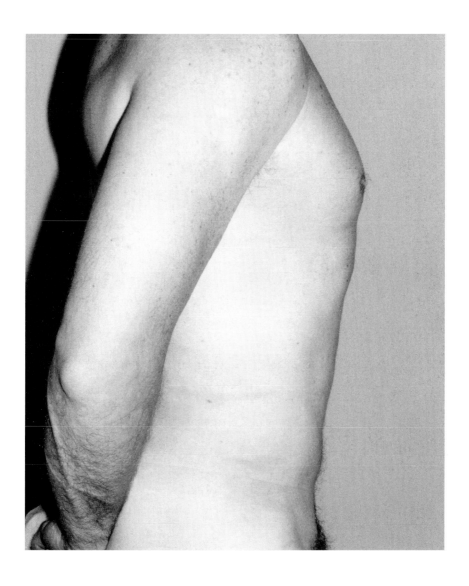

CHAPTER 42

Tummy Tucks and Mini-Tummy Tucks

This procedure removes excess skin from the stomach. The incision is designed to be hidden in bathing suit bottoms and underwear; success depends partly on how revealing those garments are (see Figure #10). While the appearance of each scar is subject to individual variation, the skin of the stomach has to be stretched and secured under a certain amount of tension in order to be tight. This may result in scars that are wider than those produced under less tension. If the surgeon closes the skin of the abdomen under too little tension, the cosmetic result may be inferior, thereby defeating the purpose of doing the surgery in the first place. Depending on the anatomy, both liposuction and a tummy tuck (several months apart) may be required to achieve the best result. In an appropriate patient, a tummy tuck produces a result that cannot be achieved with liposuction alone.

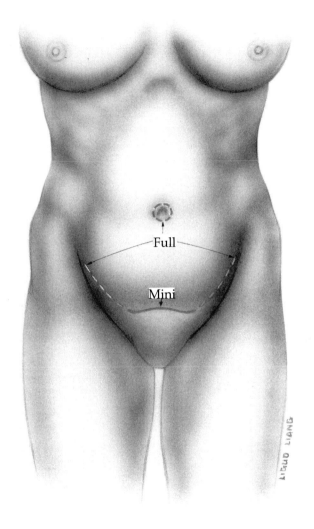

Figure 10. *Tummy Tuck / Mini-Tummy Tuck Incisions*

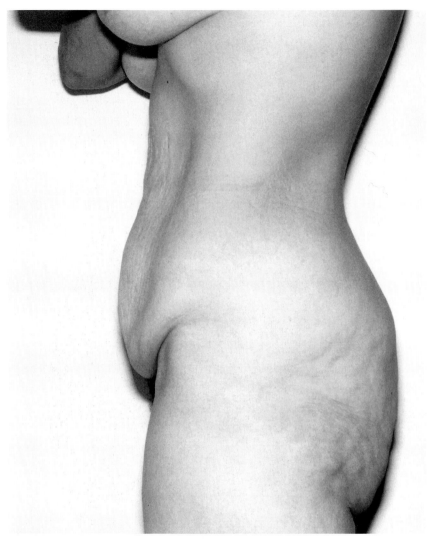

Patient Number: 61
Age: 37 years old

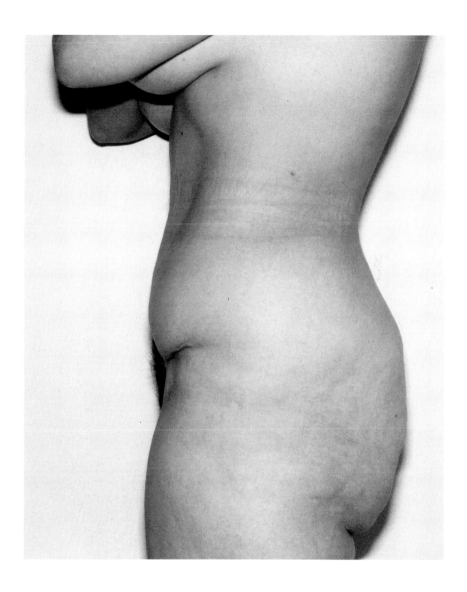

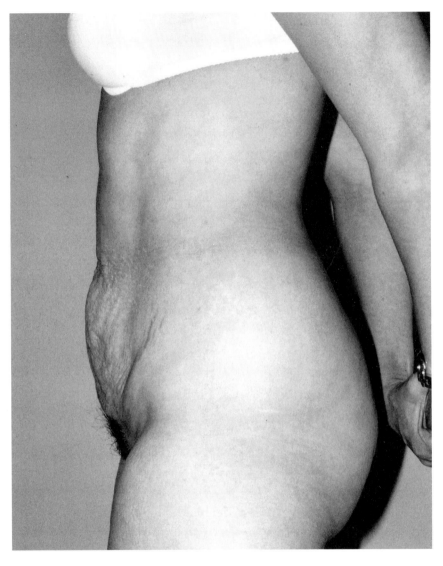

Patient Number: 62
Age: 34 years old (had liposuction at same time)

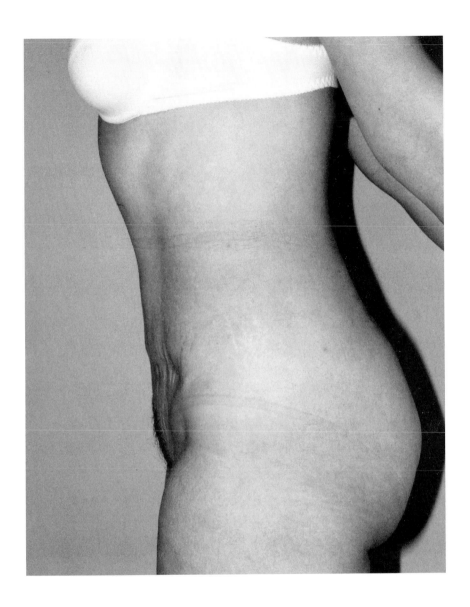

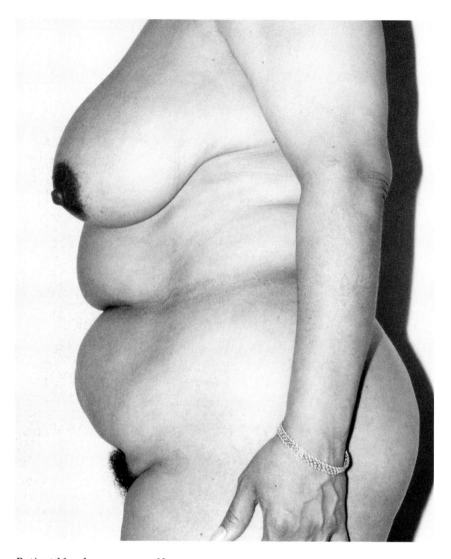

Patient Number: 63
Age: 48 years old

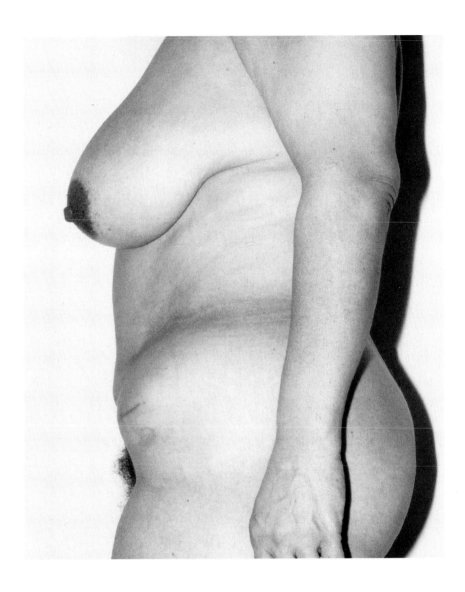

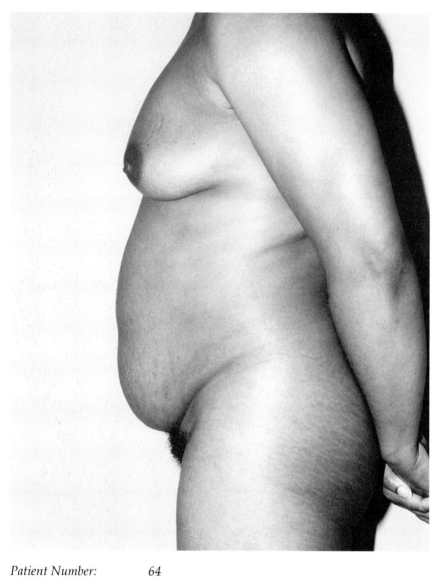

Patient Number: 64
Age: 40 years old (also had liposuction)

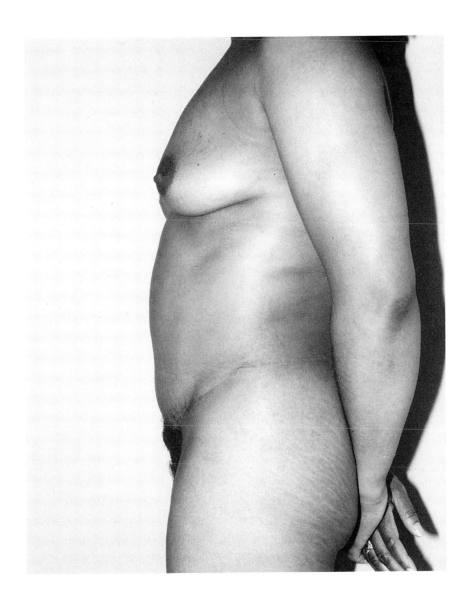

GLOSSARY

Ablation: complete removal or destruction of something (such as cancer)

Abs: the rectus abdominus muscles, the paired, vertically-oriented muscles of the abdominal wall over the stomach. The popularly termed "six-pack" is extreme development of this muscle combined with very little body fat in this region. It appears as six units (three on each side) because of the anatomic structure of the muscle and its fibrous bands, i.e., bands of connective tissue

ASAPS: The American Society for Aesthetic Plastic Surgery; www.surgery.org. Referral Service: (888) 272-7711

ASPS: The American Society of Plastic Surgeons; www.plasticsurgery.org. Referral Service: (800) 635-0635

Analgesia: lack (relief) of pain

Anesthesia: lack of sensation

Areola: the dark skin that surrounds the nipple

Aspirate: to remove fluid from a body cavity

Autoimmune diseases or reactions: a spectrum of disorders and defects in the immune system in which the body essentially rejects itself, also referred to as collagen–vascular diseases. They may be associated with impaired wound healing. The reported link between silicone gel breast implants and these disorders has not been borne out by the most recent studies

Axillary: of or referring to the underarm. Indicates the location of one of the possible incisions for breast enlargement, namely, under the arm

Biopsy: removal of tissue or fluid from the body for pathology examination

Cannula: a hollow tube used during liposuction. One end is open; the other is attached to a machine that produces the vacuum that is used to remove fat

Capsules: also called "hard breasts." This is when scar tissue forms around breast implants and hardens into a spherical shape. Implants that have formed capsules tend to appear round, ride relatively high on the breast, and do not flatten out when the woman lies down

Collagen–vascular diseases: see Autoimmune diseases

Cushing's disease or syndrome: conditions that result from or are characterized by an increase of certain steroids and may be associated with lipomas or fatty growths

Diabetes: a disorder of insulin regulation, characterized, for these purposes, by small blood vessel disease and impaired wound healing

Endoscope: a surgical instrument consisting of a long, narrow, lighted tube. It can be rigid or flexible and has a wide range of uses in medicine. It can be used to facilitate the insertion of breast implants (particularly the axillary and umbilical approaches) and for some abdominal procedures. Use of an endoscope is called Endoscopy

Endotracheal: "in the trachea" (breathing pipe); refers here to the location of the tube inserted during general anesthesia

Epinephrine: also termed adrenaline; a chemical added to the fluid injected subcutaneously during a liposuction. It constricts or tightens blood vessels, resulting in less bleeding. Also occurs naturally

Excise: to cut something out completely, e.g., a lump

Flap: a term that refers to skin (and/or muscle and other tissues) that has been largely lifted up from its surrounding area, often to be tightened and/or repositioned, as during a tummy tuck or facelift

Gynecomastia: enlargement of the male breasts

Hyperpigmented: increased pigmentation (darker in color)

Hypopigmented: decreased pigmentation (lighter in color)

Incise: to cut into something

Infragluteal: underneath the gluteal fold, i.e., the buttocks Indicates the location of one of the possible incisions for liposuction

Inframammary: underneath the breast. Indicates the location of one of the possible incisions for breast enlargement, namely, under the breast

Inhalation: the act of breathing in (inhaling). Refers to a type of anesthesia administered, particularly during general anesthesia

Intravenous: in the veins, i.e., a method of administering fluids and medications

Involutional hypomastia: small, shrunken breasts, usually as a result of pregnancy, breast feeding and/or weight loss

Laxity: looseness

Lidocaine: local anesthetic, often added to the fluid injected subcutaneously during a liposuction to decrease pain both during and after the surgery

Lipoma: a benign fatty growth, usually just under the skin

Lipoplasty: plastic surgery of fat

Liposuction: the removal of fat using a suction or vacuum technique

Lumpectomy: surgical removal of a lump, e.g., of the breast

Lupus erythematosus: an autoimmune disease

Mammography: an X-ray of the breast

Mammaplasty: plastic surgery of the breast. Breasts can be made larger (Augmentation Mammaplasty), smaller (Reduction Mammaplasty), or lifted (Mastopexy)

Mastectomy: surgical removal of an entire breast

Mastopexy: a breast lift

Pectoralis major: the major muscle of the chest, often referred to familiarly as "the pecs"

Periareolar: around the areola, which is the dark area around the nipple on a breast. Indicates the location of one of the possible incisions for breast enlargement, namely, around the lower one-third to one-half of the areola

Perioperative: around the time of the surgery

Postoperative: after surgery

Preoperative: before surgery

Prosthesis: a synthetic replacement for a body part, such as a breast or artificial limb

Quadrantectomy: surgical removal of a quadrant (a quarter), e.g., of the breast

Raynaud's disease: an autoimmune disease characterized by narrowed blood vessels

Resection: surgical removal of tissue, e.g., breast, fat, or skin

Saline: salt water, a natural liquid similar in consistency to water. It is used as a filler in breast implants

Scar revision: any of a number of surgical procedures designed to improve the appearance and/or quality of a scar

Scleroderma: an autoimmune disease characterized by tightened, scar-like skin

Seroma: serous (straw-colored) fluid that may collect under a flap, such as after a tummy tuck

Silicone: a plastic material. When formed into a gel it provides an excellent match for breast tissue and is used as a filler in breast implants. When formed into a slightly denser version, it is used as a shell for both silicone gel and saline implants. A solid form is used for implants for other parts of the body, including the chin and cheeks

Smooth: refers to a type of breast implant in which the outer surface, or shell, is smooth

Subcutaneous: under the skin

Subglandular: under the gland (such as the breast). Indicates one location for a breast implant, i.e., underneath the breast. Also termed "on top of the pectoral muscle" (this term is interchangeable with Subparenchymal)

Submuscular: under the muscle. Indicates another location for a breast implant, i.e., under the pectoralis major muscle. Technically, this term implies that the implant is also covered with portions of other chest muscles, although it is generally used interchangeably with "subpectoral"

Subparenchymal: under the tissue; in this context, directly under the breast, or above the muscle (see Subglandular)

Subpectoral: underneath the pectoralis major muscle which is the main muscle of the chest. Indicates a location for a breast implant, i.e., underneath that muscle (see Submuscular)

Textured: refers to a type of breast implant in which the outer surface, or shell, is rough and/or irregular

Tissue Expander: an inflatable implant. It is inserted under skin and tissue that need to be expanded, e.g., chest skin after a mastectomy. Once the skin is expanded over a several month period, an adequately sized breast implant replaces the expander

Tumescent: swollen hard or full of fluid. Refers to a technique of liposuction in which the tissues are injected with a large amount of fluid subcutaneously until the skin is tense and swollen

Ultrasonic Liposuction or Lipoplasty: a new technique whereby ultrasonic waves are used to "melt" and aspirate fat, after which the liquefied remnants are removed. Areas may be contoured further using traditional liposuction

Ultrasound or Ultrasonography: examination of tissues (like the breast) using a machine that emits sound waves

Umbilical: of or relating to the umbilicus (the belly button). Indicates the location of one of the possible incisions for liposuction or breast enlargement, namely, within the umbilicus

Vasoconstriction: constriction or tightening of blood vessels, an effect that decreases bleeding